"Before a heart attack or stroke 'happens' to you, read this important book. It just might save your life."

"*Before It Happens to You* presents the heart health protocol of the future. Lifestyle change is not enough to fully protect you from heart disease, even if you can really make those changes (and most of us can't). This program will protect you now."

"…This is a thoughtful, concise and clear strategy for heart health."

"Sound advice. Clearly written. Extensively researched. *Before It Happens to You* will be a valuable resource for my patients *and* my friends."

"Dr. Jonathan Sackner Bernstein offers up an 'insider's' look at the reality of what can be done to make you live longer. He takes the science that is out there and teaches you to use the information, work with your doctor and add years to your life."

"Most of us will die of heart disease, but there are ways to prevent it. This is a unique book that emphasizes maximum risk reduction, even for those who, like me, have trouble making a consistent effort at diet and exercise."

"This is an elegant and practical game plan for real health challenges. Education without admonition for both patients and doctors."

"*Before It Happens to You* has the potential to significantly and beneficially impact the field of preventive cardiology. Read it and discuss it with your doctor."

"This is a provocative patient companion in the fight against heart disease and stroke."

"*Before It Happens to You* is a totally understandable approach to long-term cardiovascular health."

—Marvin Konstam, M.D., Chief, Division of Cardiology, Tufts–New England Medical Center and President, Heart Failure Society of America

"This book provides you with the insights to truly minimize your cardiovascular risks, beyond anything found in standard guidelines."

—Michael Bristow, M.D., Ph.D., FACC, Professor of Medicine and Head, Division of Cardiology, University of Colorado Health Sciences Center

"Dr. Sackner Bernstein has taken several decades of cutting-edge heart research and developed a plan to optimize life."

—William T. Abraham, M.D., Professor of Medicine, Chief, Division of Cardiovascular Medicine, Ohio State University

"This is an unusually candid book, and certainly one of the first to reveal a major truth about preventing cardiovascular disease. It provides compelling evidence that it is the tools at your doctor's disposal—medicines used widely for a decade or longer—that can most effectively lengthen our lives and protect us from heart disease and strokes. Reading this book will have a highly positive impact on the lives of you and your family."

—Michael A. Weber, M.D., Professor of Medicine and Associate Dean, SUNY Downstate College of Medicine

"By helping us to better understand all of the medical studies, Dr. Sackner Bernstein empowers us with knowledge and enables us to help ourselves. *Before It Happens to You* also advises on how to make the interaction with our health care providers (who are only human themselves) more productive. In my opinion, *Before It Happens to You* will change your life, for the better!"

—Marc Cohen, M.D., Professor of Medicine, Director, Division of Cardiology, Newark–Beth Israel Medical Center

"A thoughtful, empowering, and provocative book. This is particularly a 'must read' for those not fortunate enough to select their parents, who have a genetic risk for developing vascular disease and thus the potential to die young."

—Alan Miller, M.D., University of Florida

"Dr. Sackner Bernstein provides a practical roadmap for the public with scientifically based strategies to minimize the risk of a heart attack or stroke. This book will save lives."

—Valentin Fuster, M.D., Ph.D., former President of the American Heart Association, President-Elect of the World Heart Federation

"An invaluable source of information for anyone who wants to take control of their health, especially women, since most women don't realize how big their risk is for serious heart disease."

—JoAnn Lindenfeld, M.D., Cardiologist

Before It Happens to You

Before It Happens to You

A Breakthrough Program for Reversing or Preventing Heart Disease

---

Jonathan Sackner Bernstein, M.D.
with Kate Kelly

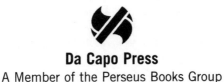

Da Capo Press
A Member of the Perseus Books Group

Designed by Jeff Williams
Set in 11.5-point Simoncini Garamond by the Perseus Books Group

Library of Congress Cataloging-in-Publication Data

Bernstein, Jonathan Sackner.
   Before it happens to you : a breakthrough program for reversing or preventing heart disease / Jonathan Sackner Bernstein, with Kate Kelly—1st ed.
      p. cm.
   ISBN 0-7382-0918-X (hardcover)
   1. Heart—Diseases—Prevention. 2. Cardiovascular system—Diseases—Prevention. I. Kelly, Kate. II. Title.
   RC672.B43 2004
   616.1'205—dc22

                                                                                    2003017459

First Da Capo Press edition 2004

Published by Da Capo Press
A Member of the Perseus Books Group
http://www.dacapopress.com

Da Capo Press books are available at special discounts for bulk purchases in the U.S. by corporations, institutions, and other organizations. For more information, please contact the Special Markets Department at the Perseus Books Group, 11 Cambridge Center, Cambridge, MA 02142, or call (800) 255-1514 or (617) 252-5298, or e-mail specialmarkets@perseusbooks.com.

Notice: No book can substitute for a clinical evaluation. This book is intended only as an informative guide for those wishing to know more about treating heart disease. In no way is this book intended to replace the advice given to you by your own physician. The ultimate decision concerning your care should be made between you and your doctor. We strongly urge you to follow his or her advice. The information in this book is offered with no guarantees on the part of the authors or Da Capo Press. The authors and Publisher disclaim all liability in connection with the use of this book.

1 2 3 4 5 6 7 8 9 / 06 05 04

For Audrey

Contents

PART THREE
Your Personalized Plan

PART FOUR
Commonsense Lifestyle Strategies

Acknowledgments

I want to express my gratitude to all those who have helped me reach this point in my personal and professional development. I have been blessed by relationships with incredible people throughout, without whom I could not have considered the prospect of writing this book. Perhaps it would be most appropriate to acknowledge the hundreds of researchers whose work form the basis for this plan. I am forever indebted to my patients, who trust me with their lives, the greatest honor anyone could receive.

But first, I wish to thank those who have contributed specifically to this book. My agent Stuart Krichevsky is so much more than a representative, advisor and negotiator; he is a trusted friend. As an editor, I could not ask for better than Marnie Cochran, whose enthusiasm is matched by her attention to detail. In her role as a co-author, Kate Kelly provided more than superb writing skills, particularly important for a first-time writer.

My wife Audrey's encouragement and support was unending, and her insights about human nature invaluable. Leonard Bernstein's feedback on the proposal and the final manuscript greatly improved the book.

Most of all, I wish to thank Seth Godin. Even if I were an experienced writer, I still don't think I could express my gratitude sufficiently. Seth was instrumental in every step I took as I became an author, starting with the idea of writing this book. He introduced me to Stuart and reviewed several versions of the manuscript, but most valuably, provided ongoing constructive criticism and support, always with generosity and tremendous insight.

I would not have been capable of writing this book if not for the many role models and colleagues who have inspired and supported me. That included role models starting with Ralph Carey, Milton Zoloth and Dwight Jaggard and colleagues during medical school and subsequent training, particularly Gordon Rubenfeld, Andy Ruzich, David Rooney and Michael Fisher. I trained under many gifted teachers, clinicians and investigators, and especially appreciate the interest taken in me by Marc Cohen, Milton Packer, Valentin Fuster, Richard Gorlin and Jose Meller. I have been privileged to work with Marvin Konstam, Douglas Mann, John McMurray and Michael Bristow. Several professional colleagues were gracious enough to review this book and provided insightful feedback, including Alan Lotvin, Red Maxwell, Marc Cohen, Marc Silver, Marvin Konstam, Alan Miller, Edward Philbin, William Abraham, Michael Weber, Clyde Yancy, Keith Aaronson, Richard Dolinar, Marrick Kukin and Hal Skopicki.

Amongst all these wonderful people, the greatest source of strength for me is my family, my wife Audrey and my incredible daughters, Sonya, Isabel and Saskia. They make the sacrifices to permit me to become the doctor that I am and made this book possible. I just hope they feel a personal sense of accomplishment from this book; because if not for them, it would never have been.

How to Use This Book

This book has three main parts:

1. The basic program: What it is and how it works
2. How to work with your doctor
3. Customizing the program for your specific needs

Part 1 explains the program, showing how quick action can decrease your chances of dying from a stroke or a heart attack by 50 percent. Your job is to immediately set up an appointment with your doctor to discuss putting the program to work for you.

Part 2 shows you how to work with your doctor to get tested and treated. Highlight the tables that are relevant to your situation and share them with your doctor. The charts will provide your doctor with the specific information needed to move forward with this program.

Part 3 offers personalized advice to people with specific conditions or in particular circumstances. After you've read about the basic program, turn to the profile chapters in Part 3 that apply to you. Whether you're a smoker or have high cholesterol, you will find a chapter that will provide you with a good game plan for what you need to do next.

In addition, suggestions for lifestyle changes are offered in Part 4. As a cardiologist, I can't help but include a brief section describing some sensible lifestyle choices you can easily make to further advance the program.

A note for readers over age 40: Start with this plan now, because the problems inside you have been going on since you were in your 20s and 30s. They've got a head start, so you've got some catching up to do.

Introduction:
The Lifestyle Myth

This book has a very simple goal: to save your life. It's why I became a doctor. For a cardiologist, life or death decisions are a daily part of the job. There isn't anything as gratifying as saving someone's life. Now I want to save *your* life.

How and Why I Developed This Plan

Sometimes being a cardiologist can be frustrating. All too often people visit a cardiologist *after* they have advanced heart disease and are too ill to be cured. Sure, cardiologists can prolong patients' lives and certainly make them feel better, but advanced heart disease is currently irreversible. Like your own doctor, I hope to read about the discovery of the cure for heart disease in this week's medical journals or hear about it at the next scientific meeting. But despite all of the advances in the fight against this country's leading cause of death, the overall progress is still slow.

My recent breakthrough, which I will share with you in this book, isn't the discovery of a new gene; it was a lot simpler than that. What I've discovered from hundreds of scientific studies by thousands of researchers is a very straightforward idea: If you start treatment *before* you develop any symptoms of heart disease, you'll live longer.

I spend a lot of time lecturing to other doctors from all over the world, and to prepare I do a lot of reading. This has given me an opportunity to study all the evidence available, and over time I have found reason for hope. What I realized was this: Heart disease starts at least 20 or 30 years before it becomes life threatening, and well before symptoms develop. It is reversible in these early stages. I learned through my clinical work that I could save more lives, actually spare people from heart disease, if I could start reaching patients earlier—early enough to encourage them to be aggressively screened and treated before the disease takes hold.

Most people respond to this news by saying, "But I already *am* screened for heart disease. Every time I go to the doctor, I have my blood pressure and cholesterol checked. I'm fine."

This is not enough. Too often the medical community lets patients experience major crises (heart attacks, strokes or arrhythmias) and then acts, instead of starting treatment when blood pressure and cholesterol begin to rise. Unfortunately, once there has been a "cardiac event" of some type, the underlying heart disease is so advanced that some patients become sicker and die within only a few years. On average, a quarter of men and more than a third of women die within a year of their first heart attack. Because heart attacks occur in the young and middle-aged as well as in older people, this can mean a person's lifespan is greatly reduced.

So your doctor said you are okay. Yes, you may be okay *according to government guidelines.* What the layperson doesn't know is that these standards that are set for acceptable blood pressure and cholesterol levels are not written with your best interest as the primary consideration. They are written with the cost-benefit ratio for society in mind: If a safe therapy reduces the risk of dying young by only 10 percent, it may be too costly for the government to justify it as a general recommendation for the entire population, despite its potential to markedly prolong life.

As written, the government guidelines recommend levels that bring people to "low risk," but not to "lowest risk." While many doctors understand this difference and treat people optimally, studies show that most do not. Even doctors who do understand the difference may not have extra time to spend on patient education.

Don't worry. I'm not going to recommend a battery of expensive tests. The Before It Happens Plan, as I call it, has a simple foundation based on more rigorous interpretation of the results of standard tests—tests without risk to you. Screening for high blood pressure and increased cholesterol levels is a good start. But it's the interpretation of these tests that is so important in reducing risk. As an example, the results of your cholesterol profile tests should be much better than the current guidelines recommend if you want to minimize your risk. I'll show you how to ask for treatment to achieve optimal goals, not just acceptable ones.

As I've continued to travel, doing presentations for colleagues, I've been sharing the plan with them over the course of the last year. Most of the doctors who hear about the plan do one thing first: They put themselves and their families on it. Once you understand why you are in danger of suffering a heart attack or stroke, you'll realize why you need to be treated with the medicines in this plan and what you can do to keep your own life free from risk.

Few of Us Can Change Our Lifestyle

There are three kinds of people with heart disease. One realizes the importance of eating well and exercising regularly, and has followed this healthy lifestyle before developing symptomatic heart disease. Already living the healthy lifestyle, there isn't much room for improvement.

Another is more typical, people who are not nearly as healthy as they could be. It would be terrific if everyone were disciplined enough to improve their lifestyle, changing 40- or 50-year-old habits, keeping their heart as healthy as possible. But not all of us can. If you fit this profile, it's not that you're lazy or slothful—you're human. When 400 doctors were asked to grade the ability of their patients to change their lifestyles, the average grade was D+, so don't feel too bad.

Maybe you are the third type, the rare person who can adopt a healthy lifestyle. That would be great. But lifestyle modification is not enough; it helps only modestly. It is worth every effort to reduce your risk even a little, but it is sobering to see how small the effect of lifestyle change is in comparison with the medicines of this plan.

Despite the data, the myth continues to spread that lifestyle modification is the way to protect yourself from the risks of heart disease. You can see evidence of this myth in all the health books for sale, or consider what your doctor tells you. But the truth is that while improving your lifestyle will help, it's not nearly as effective as the medicines in this program.

That's why I will not give you much advice about why or how you should change your lifestyle. The plan I'm presenting in this book is something you can actually do—without willpower or side effects. It's a plan that will help you stay alive for a long time, whether or not you can change your lifestyle.

The heart of the plan is simple: a combination of tested, safe drugs that you take every day. Some require a prescription, and some are as simple as aspirin. If used the right way, these medicines have been shown to actually reverse heart disease and prevent heart attacks, strokes and premature death.

The medicines in this plan have excellent safety records and are safer than most arthritis medications and many common antibiotics. In fact, they've been shown to be far safer than the untested vitamins that you may be taking every day without even thinking about them.

I will show you how these medicines can reduce your risk of dying young, typically adding years to your life. Of course, you need to be evaluated individually by your doctor, even before deciding to take aspirin regularly. You will be able to achieve optimal health by using a customized mix of the following medicines:

- Aspirin
- Statins
- Beta-blockers
- ACE inhibitors

Some people may need a diuretic as well, if their blood pressure is high. That's it. No expensive, intricate diets, no new rigorous exercise plans. *If you can swallow a pill, you can prolong your life.*

There are no brand-new medicines in this plan and no blockbuster technological breakthroughs. Instead you will be prescribed older medications whenever possible. As a researcher, my career is focused on finding new drugs and procedures. As a clinician, my practice is to rely on older medicines with established track records. For one thing, they are often cheaper. But more importantly, they are better tested on huge populations so we know their safety and effectiveness with great precision.

Using this plan, you will keep yourself healthy and alive, whether or not you are able to change your lifestyle.

PART 1

Simple, Safe and Scientific:
The Breakthrough Program

CHAPTER 1

You're Probably Going to Die from Heart Disease

*"Be careful about reading health books.
You may die of a misprint."*

MARK TWAIN

HEART DISEASE STARTS MUCH EARLIER THAN YOU THINK. You're probably suffering from it right now. In your 20s and 30s, little balls of fat started forming in the walls of your arteries. You can't feel them and your doctor can't find them by any standard tests—not a stress test, not even a fancy CAT scan or any of the new technologies—but they're there, and they can cause trouble without warning. If one of these fat deposits were to burst open, you would have a heart attack or drop dead suddenly.

Consider these facts. When the hearts of soldiers killed in Korea and Vietnam were examined during autopsies, scientists made a startling discovery: Even though the average age of the soldiers was 22, 20 percent of them already had *significant* plaques in the arteries of their hearts. These plaques (fatty deposits in the walls of the arteries) would have grown, blocking oxygen and nutrients from getting to the heart muscle. Or, they could have ruptured and abruptly stopped blood flow, leading to death. This was confirmed by investigators at the University of Kentucky who found that 75 percent of young trauma victims (age 14 to 35) had significant heart disease and did not even realize it.

Your arteries also are getting stiffer, a process that will lead to high blood pressure in more than half of American adults. We know that treating high blood pressure prevents heart attacks, strokes and kidney failure. We have the tools (the medicines in this program) to radically improve your odds. Yet the medical establishment continues to ignore the scientific proof. While doctors are advised to keep patients' blood pressure under 140/90, a person's risk is cut in half when blood pressure is under 115/75. I'll show you the data and how to put it to work.

You may be thinking you're too young and too healthy to worry about having a heart attack. Unfortunately, science has a harsh message for you. You are at far greater risk than you realize. As your age increases, so does your risk. Most people in their 50s have abnormal blood pressure (the average is 125/80). If you are in your 40s, you have a 70 percent chance of having significant plaque building up in your coronary arteries. If you are over 50, you have an 85 percent chance.

By 45, We *All* Have Heart Disease

To understand why this plan, the Before It Happens Plan, is so important, it helps to understand why heart disease is so difficult to treat. At the onset of heart disease, the abnormalities in your heart and blood vessels are small, hard to detect but easy to treat. Unfortunately, doctors are currently trained only to detect and treat disease once it is

---

The Definition of High Blood Pressure
....

Even doctors don't agree on the definition of high blood pressure. Traditionally, if your pressure were above 140/90 (measured more than once), you would have hypertension (high blood pressure). Multiple studies over the past 50 years define abnormal blood pressure as higher than 115/75 or 120/80. Anything higher is associated with an increased risk of heart attack, stroke or early death.

more advanced—and far less reversible. This is why the plan focuses primarily on healthy people with less severe heart disease. If you have more advanced heart disease, it will still reduce your risk by 30 to 50 percent. The less advanced your heart disease is, the more years the plan can add to your life, so that an average 50-year-old could live 10, 15 or 20 years longer without a heart attack or stroke. The truth is, even though many of us will die from heart disease, we typically feel fine until we do, but that's just because the symptoms usually don't show up until it's too late.

So, if we can't successfully test for the early stages of heart disease, should we just wait until it becomes noticeable and hard to treat? I don't think so. Rather than waiting to treat heart disease until after you are at risk of dying prematurely, start now, while it is easier and more effective. I'm proposing that no matter your age, if you have any evidence of cardiovascular disease, you need to start this program *now*.

What if your blood pressure, cholesterol and weight are already optimal? If you are nearing 50, your risk is high anyway. You have 30 years of cholesterol-filled plaques building up in the walls of your arteries. A man has at least a 1 in 50 chance of having a heart attack in the next 10 years. A woman's risk of a heart attack is lower, and doesn't rise above 1 in 100 until around 55 (around menopause). So while a woman is more likely to be diagnosed with breast cancer in midlife than to suffer a heart attack (or die from one), many more women develop significant cardiovascular disease in their 50s than are diagnosed with breast cancer. By the time women reach their 60s, they are increasingly likely to suffer a heart attack or stroke because of the natural tendency for the disease to worsen over time. Because the medicines are so safe, treatment is beneficial for women as well.

We hear about it every day: people suffering a stroke, a heart attack or worse, dropping dead in the prime of life. No warning, no reason, not even any sign of disease. Sometimes the victim is a friend or relative, other times a celebrity or politician. The most frequent cause? Heart disease.

**You need the Before It Happens Plan
if you have any of these characteristics:**
••

- Elevated blood pressure (above 115/75)
- Elevated LDL cholesterol (above 100) or total cholesterol (above 160)
- Low HDL cholesterol (men less than 40, women less than 50)
- Have a first-degree relative with heart disease (parent, sibling or child)
- Are a current or past smoker
- Are overweight (more than 10 percent above ideal body weight)
- Are around age 50 or older, or postmenopausal
- Have diabetes, are insulin-resistant, or have borderline or diet-controlled diabetes

---

And as hard as it is to believe, you're probably going to die from heart disease, too. That's no misprint. Each year, more than half of all deaths in America are caused by heart disease. That's more than all forms of cancer *combined.* Cardiovascular disease, which includes diseases of the heart and blood vessels, is also the number one cause of death and permanent disability for people between 40 and 65. A million Americans suffer a heart attack every year—and 30 percent of them die suddenly and unexpectedly before ever making it to the hospital.

Your doctor is working hard to make sure you're not going to be one of those statistics. Based on your medical condition and standard tables of statistics, patients are classified as high, moderate or low risk. Low-risk patients—those with less than a 10 percent risk of heart disease or cardiovascular disease over the next 10 years—generally receive no medication but are counseled to adopt a healthier lifestyle. Your doctor will send you on your way, as the guidelines dictate.

Changing your lifestyle is your responsibility, and if you want to get better, you need to do it yourself.

People at higher risk may be given some medication, but medical professionals tend to rely on part of the work being done by the patient. They undermedicate, assuming people who have gotten a "wake-up call" in the form of being diagnosed with high blood pressure or elevated cholesterol will mend their ways and alter their eating and exercise habits or finally quit smoking.

While this may seem like a reasonable approach, there are three flaws inherent in this strategy. Studies prove that few people with such a wake-up call actually do change their lifestyle. Consider your own situation. You know you would be better off with a healthier lifestyle, but do you exercise regularly, maintain an ideal weight and really eat a well-balanced diet (without any junk food)? I know how hard it is. I know that I should go swimming on my way to work, but there always seems to be a project to do or a meeting to attend. A healthy lifestyle is not so easy to integrate into your family life and career.

The second flaw is that our national guidelines aren't stringent enough. The government must base its recommendation on the total amount to be spent relative to the benefit of that investment for society (the cost-benefit ratio). Because it would be too costly to society to have everyone—even lower risk patients—on blood pressure and cholesterol-lowering medications, the government sets standards that are a compromise, reserving more aggressive treatment for those at higher risk and setting goals to help everyone a little, which is much more affordable than helping everyone a lot. That's why you need to be your own advocate.

The third flaw is that even if you could intensively change your lifestyle, this would provide only a fraction of the benefit that you would realize from the Before It Happens Plan. The medical therapies in this breakthrough plan can cut your risk by as much as 50 to 75 percent. The ideal would be to realize the benefits of both lifestyle change and medical therapies.

When the medical standards were first established for the prevention and treatment of cardiovascular disease, there weren't many safe and effective treatment options available, so a low-risk patient could have been described as someone whose risk from the disease was about the same (or lower) than the risk from the treatment. However, over the past 20 to 30 years, all that has changed. Now we have safe, effective treatments for heart disease, medicines that are so safe that more low-risk patients deserve to be treated. A doctor who does not prescribe these medicines widely may be placing you in unnecessary danger (even if you are a low-risk patient).

I met a 39-year-old woman in my hospital emergency room when she suffered a heart attack. Just two weeks earlier, she'd been to see her doctor, complaining that she was worn out trying to keep up with her kids. The doctor took her symptoms seriously and ordered a stress test, which is standard practice. The test results were normal; but despite having "borderline" high blood pressure, she was sent home with advice to change her lifestyle. I would have treated her according to the Before It Happens Plan and started her on an aspirin, beta-blocker and ACE inhibitor that day. If her blood test showed an LDL cholesterol level above 100, I would add a statin as well. If her symptoms were not better in a couple of days, and no other cause was evident, I would have referred her for a cardiac catheterization. (This is a test in which catheters are inserted through the arteries in your groin or arm and advanced to the arteries of your heart, where X-ray films can be taken to detect the presence of blockages that may require an angioplasty or stent.)

Unfortunately, without any treatment initiated, she was in my hospital two weeks later, having an emergency angioplasty to open two coronary artery blockages. The procedure went well, but a major part of her heart had already died as a result of this heart attack, and she faces a future where it is unlikely that she will lead a normal life.

Consider this risk comparison: A 57-year-old woman with high blood pressure, treated successfully as defined by the standard guidelines, has a 1 in 200 chance of death over the next year, while a 48-

year-old man with borderline blood pressure has a risk of 1 in 167. If you were either of these two people, and you implemented this plan, the risk would be 1 in 1,000—an 80 percent reduction in risk.

Whether you are low, moderate or high risk, the data are clear: The Before It Happens Plan can reduce your risk of dying from heart disease. The standard recommendations may be good for society, but for you, a person at risk of a heart attack or premature death, they're more like playing Russian roulette.

Why It's Important to Pay Attention Now

To be effective, treatment must start when the disease is in its early stages. This is the goal of the Before It Happens Plan, since the plaques in the walls of your arteries can rupture unpredictably, triggering a heart attack, stroke or worse. Treating early gives two major advantages over the standard practice of waiting until the disease is more advanced. First, earlier in the development of the disease, the abnormalities are easier to reverse. Second, for some people, heart disease becomes evident in a rather unsettling way—they drop dead without warning (sudden cardiac death). Certainly, anyone would want to make sure that treatment starts before that is about to happen, and this is no small problem, as 300,000 Americans suffer sudden cardiac death each year.

My friend Howard was almost one of them. Howard is a 48-year-old academic internist—a doctor who teaches doctors. I shared my research for this book with him and told him about how I treat my patients aggressively for heart disease. Howard showed more than casual interest.

It turns out that he jogs a few miles a day, doesn't smoke and has pretty good cholesterol and blood pressure readings. He has no family history of heart disease. All the traditional measures would put him on the lower end of the risk scale, and he would not be receiving treatment.

A few months ago, Howard decided to ask his doctor about the "heartburn" he'd experience after running. It turned out that Howard had such severe blockages in his arteries that he needed to have an invasive procedure to install a stent, a small tube designed to keep his arteries open. Here's a smart, healthy doctor who didn't know he was dying from heart disease until it was almost too late.

Don't wait until it's too late for you.

The Plan: Simple, Safe and Scientific

The Before It Happens Plan is *simple.* You are at risk of dying from cardiovascular disease. This plan would typically cut your risk in half.

This plan is *safe.* Could you have a side effect or allergic reaction to one of the medicines? Yes, but you are much more likely to suffer a heart attack or stroke. Life is a set of choices, and I think you want to take the path of lowest possible risk. That means this plan is for you. Two of the medicines are so safe that one is over-the-counter (aspirin) and another is being switched to over-the-counter in the United Kingdom (statins). The other two are available only by prescription, because blood tests and measurement of your blood pressure are necessary to determine the proper dosages.

This plan is *scientific* because the proof is well established throughout the medical literature. The scientific evidence should persuade your doctor. It establishes beyond doubt that this program reflects optimal care. In the next chapter, while reviewing the tools of the plan, you will see charts that will prove useful in your process of enlightening your doctor about the merits of the plan.

With all the money the drug companies spend on advertising, why aren't they promoting this plan? In order to promote a drug, a pharmaceutical company needs to work with the FDA and do extensive testing. Tests can take a decade or more and cost many millions of dollars. Only after the testing is done and approved is the drug approved for sale, but with an important limitation: The drug can only be promoted for precisely what it was tested for. Your doctor, of course, can prescribe the drug for any use he or she desires. (That's how botox treatments caught on—the drug wasn't approved for wrinkle removal, but it has been found to be safe enough to be marketed for other uses.)

To market this combination of medicines to the general public as a heart disease prevention strategy, the drug companies would have to spend hundreds of millions of dollars over many years on research studies testing each of the possible combinations. They can't do that, because no company manufactures all of the individual types of medicines in the plan, and each of these drugs is so old that they couldn't possibly make the money back that they would need to invest. So it's up to your doctor to tell you about how these safe drugs can be used to protect you.

Doctors at Queen Mary's School of Medicine and Dentistry in London made the case for their own version of the Before It Happens Plan. They studied the effects of a theoretical medicine called a "polypill" that would contain the four medicines of the plan, plus a diuretic and folic acid. They advocated that everyone in the world over 55 should take such a pill, because their analysis estimated an 88 percent reduction in cardiovascular disease. Although there are insufficient data to support the inclusion of folic acid, and the impact could be better for you if the components and their dosages could be individualized, the doctors at Queen Mary's are the first to advocate such a plan to doctors in the medical literature. This book is the first to bring the plan for optimal prevention to you, the patient.

Implementing the Plan

You've already made the commitment to read this book, so I know you want to optimize your health. In the second section of this book, I will show you how to talk to your doctor about this plan.

You are the boss when it comes to your health; your doctor is your consultant.

Your doctor should be your educator and advisor. You are in charge of the overall strategy, and then your doctor should implement treatment consistent with your goals. This may not be feasible in a life-threatening emergency, but it is the ideal approach. To do this, you must understand the "rules" of communication, which will be explained in Part 2. These rules outline the easiest way to talk to your doctor about your health.

CHAPTER 2

The Workings of the Cardiovascular System

"No one wants to know how *it works, only* that *it works."*

THE MATRIX RELOADED

IF YOU'VE READ OTHER HEALTH BOOKS, YOU MAY THINK YOU already understand the basic workings of the cardiovascular system well enough to skip this chapter—but don't. This chapter describes the changes to your system caused by high cholesterol and high blood pressure, so you can understand what is happening to your body— then you'll want to do what you can to reduce your risks.

At first glance, the cardiovascular system is a simple one, with a pump moving blood through a series of pipes (arteries and veins) to supply the body with its metabolic needs. The heart muscle pumps with incredible endurance. It beats 70 times a minute all day, every day. By the time you reach the age of 70, your heart has pumped 2,575,440,000 times. The heart serves at the mercy of the vascular system, primarily the arteries that supply nutrients to it and to all vital organs. In the heart, there are three main arteries that supply blood to the heart muscle, each of which is only about 3 to 6 mm in diameter at its widest.

In actuality, the cardiovascular system is incredibly complex, with layer after layer of safeguards preserving its function in response to any conceivable need. To ensure your survival, most of these mechanisms that so efficiently support short-term stability do so at the

13

> Cholesterol and blood pressure problems account for more than half of the risk that you face. The more effectively you can reverse them, the more dramatically this program will reduce your risk.

expense of long-term dysfunction. Cholesterol metabolism and blood pressure control are the two processes that your body masks particularly well, with no evidence of any problems until the damage is pretty advanced.

Cholesterol and the Problems It Creates

Cholesterol is a vital part of the structure of every cell in your body and an important building block for hormones and other chemicals your body makes. And while people worry about how their diet affects their cholesterol level, few people realize that the liver makes most of the cholesterol in your body—it makes more cholesterol than your body needs. Reducing cholesterol from your diet has a relatively minor impact, although eating more cholesterol can be especially dangerous.

Cholesterol floats through your blood in two primary forms: as a low-density lipoprotein (LDL, or the "bad" cholesterol), delivering what is needed, and as a high-density lipoprotein (HDL, the "good" cholesterol), removing the excess. Cholesterol also circulates in a form called triglyceride. A high triglyceride level is bad, but not as bad as an elevated LDL level. (Triglyceride plays a relatively minor role in the health of your heart and blood vessels, but if the level is very high, it can increase your risk and also interfere with the machines used to measure the amount of LDL in the blood.)

> Your liver makes more than three times as much cholesterol as you eat— every day, no matter what.

As the LDL circulates, much of it enters the inner lining of your arteries, forming little bumps called plaques. This is the start of cardiovascular disease, and believe it or not, this begins in your 20s. Since cholesterol is not needed in the walls of the artery, your body tries to digest and remove it. The process is well suited as a short-term protective mechanism, but causes problems long-term. It's as if the body is taking this toxic product (cholesterol) and putting it in bins and burying it, without a plan for what to do if the bins leak or are unearthed.

This cholesterol buildup activates your immune system, and all sorts of cells respond, entering your plaque by burrowing through the cap that lines its surface. To get in, these immune cells release enzymes that create small openings between the cells lining the plaque, through which the immune cells pass. Once the immune cells are inside the plaque, they work to clear the cholesterol. Immune cells release chemicals to help digest the cholesterol, but one type, called free radicals, can damage other cells in a way that makes the plaques more vulnerable to rupture.

Because free radicals can damage normal cells, the body tries to limit the amount of these toxic chemicals that are produced. By altering the structure of cholesterol, the stimulus for free radical production is markedly reduced. Unfortunately, this modified cholesterol cannot be cleared from the wall of the artery and causes the plaque to grow. This is the equivalent of a growing pile of toxic waste–filled drums.

Plaques usually take on one of two characteristics: either they become big enough to block flow (what doctors call obstructing lesions) or they remain small, fat filled and inflamed (vulnerable plaques). If your body is able to form a thick cap over the plaque and stop the immune cells from invading, the plaque becomes a non-threatening stable scar in the vessel wall. Encouraging this process is one of the major targets of this program.

Figure 2.1 shows a segment of an artery wall. In your 20s and 30s, small amounts of cholesterol start to deposit in the walls of the arteries, covered by thin caps. By midlife, in your 40s or 50s, the cholesterol deposits have formed plaques with caps over them that are vulnerable to rupture. When that happens, a blood clot starts to form. If the rupture in the cap is big or the plaque is particularly inflamed, the clot rapidly grows and blocks the vessel opening, leading to a heart attack, stroke or sudden death. If you're lucky, the blood clot will remain small, eventually becoming calcified. Calcified plaques can remain small or grow, but in either case become less likely to rupture. (See Figure 2.1.)

The obstructing lesions are the ones most likely to cause symptoms (such as chest pain or discomfort, shortness of breath or decreased exercise capacity), both with daily activities and during stress tests. These lesions don't usually cause heart attacks, and are the types of lesions that become calcified over time, making them easier to detect with sophisticated CAT scans. When you have these lesions, you can have them fixed using angioplasty, stents or bypass surgery if medicines cannot control the symptoms adequately.

If you have obstructing lesions, you also have vulnerable plaques. Most likely, you have vulnerable plaques without the obstructing ones (see Figure 2.2). The plaques are called vulnerable because they are the ones at risk of rupturing, which may result in a heart attack or stroke.

Remember the enzymes the immune cells release to enter the plaques? Sometimes the cracks burst open, exposing the cholesterol deposits and immune cells within the plaque to the circulation, and immediately a blood clot starts to form. Within seconds, the clot can completely block the flow of blood. This is the beginning of a heart attack (or stroke if in an artery leading to the brain). For each minute that it takes to open that artery up again, your risk of dying increases.

Why Less-than-Perfect Blood Pressure Is Dangerous

A single pumping action constitutes a heartbeat. When the heart muscle contracts (the actual beat), it pumps blood out of the heart, sending out a pressure wave through your arteries. The walls expand as the blood flows forward, creating what is called *systolic pressure.* When the heart muscle relaxes before the next heartbeat, this allows the blood to fill up the heart again, and this is known as *diastolic pressure.*

Plaques Develop by Our 30s and Start to Rupture in Our 50s

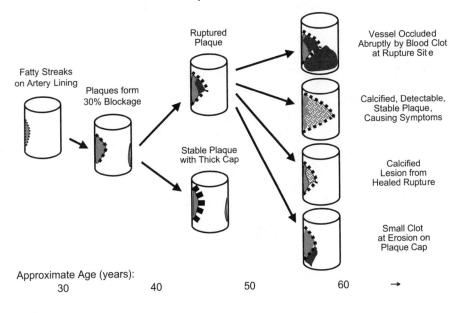

Figure 2.1 Without any symptoms, cholesterol deposits in your arteries starting as a young adult and gets progressively worse over several decades.

In this figure, the tubes represent one section of a coronary artery, the blood vessels in your heart. Plaques of lipid, often with inflammatory cells are shown in gray. Over decades, your body tries to limit their growth by making a lining of cells and scar tissue on top, and this "cap" is shown as a dotted black line.

If your plaques are covered by thick caps, they will become less likely to rupture. The medicines in this plan promote thick, strong caps and more stable plaques, less likely to rupture.

In general, by middle age, we'll have some caps that are stable and others prone to burst open. When this plaque rupture occurs, the inflamed fatty plaques are exposed to the blood, causing the formation of a blood clot, shown in black, the first step in a heart attack and possibly sudden death (or a stroke when this happens in an artery in the brain).

In some cases, the rupture is small and the blood clot seals it without blocking blood flow in the artery. Over time, calcium deposits within these plaques (shown as stippled in the figure). These calcified lesions don't usually cause a heart attack because they harden and don't rupture easily, as opposed to the soft fatty plaques.

Over 70% of People Without Apparent Cardiovascular Disease Have Coronary Artery Plaques by Their 40s

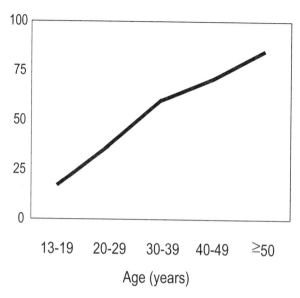

Figure 2.2 To know for sure whether your coronary arteries have plaques in them, you would need the test performed by the cardiologists at the Cleveland Clinic in this study.

First patients underwent a coronary angiogram, where small tubes are inserted into the arteries in your groin, passed up into the heart and its arteries, and pictures are taken using x-rays. That is the standard part, which is the best test to detect plaques that are blocking most of an artery, but the test can't find the small lesions very accurately (the ones blocking only 30% of the blood vessel).

Next, another catheter was inserted into the arteries of the heart, one with a small ultrasound machine on its tip to allow it to take pictures of the artery from the inside. This is a test that most "invasive" cardiologists can perform, but it is not nearly as safe or easy as a plain old angiogram.

Their findings are scary. These people were not suspected of having heart disease, and in general had normal echocardiograms and probably would have had normal stress tests. Despite this, the proportion of people with coronary artery disease is astounding 71 percent of people in their 40s and 85 percent of those in their 50s stress test, or would have.

These are the two numbers used to measure your blood pressure. If either number of your blood pressure is above 115/75, your risk is higher than it should be.

Your doctor may talk to you about having prehypertension (between 115/75 and 140/90) or grade 1, 2 or 3 hypertension. The higher the grade, the worse your risk and the more urgently you need treatment. You don't need to know the definitions of the grades, just that a higher blood pressure or a higher blood pressure grade means your risk is higher.

As you age, your arteries become less flexible and the heart has to push harder to get the blood through, which leads to increased blood pressure. The change can be mild at first, and in some cases, a small change escapes your doctor's notice because neither you nor your doctor thinks much about a single blood pressure reading in the 125/80 range, since this is within the "standard" normal range. However, if you used to have blood pressure that was lower, for example, 110/70 a reading of 125/80 indicates that you are in the early stages of having high blood pressure.

A rise in your blood pressure is not controlled like a light switch—you do not go from years of having a blood pressure of 110/70 to 150/90 overnight. This process is gradual and subtle, taking place over a period of years. Early in the process of developing high blood pressure, as your pressure starts to rise, the cause is functional and not due to structural changes in your blood vessels. The functional problems are more readily reversed than the structural changes that follow, making this the ideal time to implement this plan.

The increase in the pressure your doctor measures is only one part of what is changing, but the others are not so easy to measure. Normally, your body controls blood flow precisely, but as the blood vessels start to malfunction, your system becomes less efficient at it. That means that exercising muscles may not get all the blood they need, and more importantly, vital organs might not either.

If you do not address your blood pressure problems in this early stage, your heart and arteries start to change structurally, making the changes less reversible and impairing further your body's ability to distribute blood flow. This puts greater demands on your heart, adding to your risk of a heart attack or stroke.

Your arteries have to figure out the way to compensate with the increased pressure at a time when they are becoming less and less flexible. Inside the walls of the arteries, the muscle cells start to grow, which we call hypertrophy, just as the muscle cells in your arms and legs do when you exercise (this growth is the way cells compensate for the extra work they have to do). While this helps the arteries tolerate the higher pressure, they become even more rigid, raising blood pressure more and stimulating muscle hypertrophy further. The cycle drives up the blood pressure and adds extra stress to your heart. In response, the heart muscle cells start to grow as well. Hypertrophy of the heart is a sign that your cardiovascular system is not doing well and that you are at even higher risk of strokes and premature death.

The stiffening and dysfunction of your blood vessels become more prominent in your 40s and 50s, the same time when the plaques in your arteries become more prominent. The higher pressure markedly increases the likelihood of plaque rupture.

Though most doctors would tell you that you have acceptable blood pressure, your risk actually increases as soon as your pressure is above 115/75. With the safe medicines available today, the risk of abnormal blood pressure is higher than the risk of the treatment, even if your doctor tells you that your blood pressure is only in the prehypertension or borderline range. The medicines in this program restore normal function and can reverse much of the structural damage, and in doing so reduce your risk.

What Other Risks Predispose You to Heart Disease?

Your risk of a heart attack or dying increases when tests show that your:

- LDL cholesterol > 100
- HDL cholesterol is low (< 40 for a man, < 50 for a woman)
- Blood pressure > 115/75
- HgA$_{1c}$* > 6% (for diabetics)
- Heart chambers are enlarged or weak
- Homocysteine > 5
- C-Reactive Protein (CRP) > 1

I am not a fan of the way the medical establishment addresses the classic risk factors. I know that abnormal cholesterol, high blood pressure, smoking, diabetes, a family history of premature heart disease and being a man all predispose you to cardiovascular disease. But just look at how many people have heart attacks or die suddenly without any of these classic risk factors. I could flip a coin and be almost as accurate a predictor (only slightly more than half of heart attack victims had classic risk factors).

If your doctor says you have "positive" risk factors for heart disease, that may help you understand you're at risk, but the problem is that the definition of "positive" is arbitrary. For example, you are considered hypertensive with a blood pressure above 140/90, but we know that your risk of a heart attack is higher even if your blood pressure is just above 115/75.

Or, you are considered at greater risk if your father had a heart attack before he was 55; but what if your father went to bed the night before his 55th birthday and woke up with the symptoms of a heart attack? Should that have different meaning for you, depending on whether he woke up before or after midnight? Strictly speaking, that would make the difference between having a "positive" family history or not. The risk is greater when the heart attack occurred younger, but is still relevant even if your father's heart attack was at the age of 62.

---

*Many doctors use the terms HgA$_{1c}$ and glycohemoglobin interchangeably. Although they are closely related, normal values for glycohemoglobin are slightly higher.

The traditional approach is to list the risks for a given individual and address those that are modifiable. We can't change some things, such as your age or your genes (your family history), and these factors are ignored in the decision making process. Therapy starts with lifestyle modification, but we know the problems with that strategy: few can do it, and even when someone can, it lowers risk only a little bit.

That is why these risks fall into three categories: those that *scientifically can't be changed,* those that *you won't change* and those that are *easily modifiable* (see the chart below). Even those factors that aren't modifiable should affect the way other targets are treated. For example, if you have a history of heart disease in your family, you want a doctor to treat you more aggressively.

Part 2 shows you how to help your doctor look at the data with an open mind. From there it will be simple for you to get the optimal treatment for these modifiable risks, and reverse your cardiovascular disease.

Categories of Risk		
Scientifically Can't Change	**You Won't Change**	**Easily Modifiable**
Your genes (family history)	Smoking	Blood pressure
Race	Sedentary lifestyle	Cholesterol
Gender	Obesity/overweight	Diabetes control
Age		

Major Cardiovascular Disorders

The remainder of this chapter will provide brief definitions and descriptions for the major and common cardiovascular disorders. If you are diagnosed with a problem that does not appear below, ask your doctor if your condition has any other names, or show him or her this list. If your problem is not on this list, then this program is not for you.

Angina: This term describes chest pain, pressure or discomfort that originates in the heart muscle. It comes as a result of inadequate blood supply to the heart muscles, generally during exertion, and is relieved by rest. Angina occurs when a plaque in one of the coronary arteries is big enough to block blood flow almost completely; certainly enough to prevent the needed increase in blood flow during exertion. The discomfort varies from mild to severe. It may be limited to a constricting feeling in the center of the chest, or the pain may radiate down one or both arms. It may feel like heartburn, or you could feel it in your jaw, neck or even your back. The symptoms can be even less typical in women, as I describe in Chapter 15. If the pain is not relieved after resting for 15 minutes, it may be a sign of heart attack. Ask your doctor what to do if you experience angina: Should you call 9-1-1, should you wait until the next day to call the doctor's office or are there other steps to consider? If you have not discussed this with your doctor and have any chest pains, call your doctor right away. This isn't a symptom to ignore.

Atherosclerosis: This disorder comes about when the arteries narrow and harden because of an accumulation of cholesterol and other fatty substances in the walls of the arteries. Those who are lucky enough to have warning symptoms may experience chest pain or discomfort (angina). This condition is often symptomless; people don't realize they have it until they experience a heart attack or stroke. Suffice it to say, we all have this by middle age—autopsies done on most people who die in middle age show atherosclerosis to be prevalent.

Arrhythmias: An arrhythmia is an irregularity in your heartbeat caused by disturbances to the heart's electrical system. These irregularities can be from something relatively harmless, like too much coffee, or they can be a sign of cardiovascular disease. The sensation of awareness of your heart beat is called *palpitations.* In general, palpitations with no other symptoms in someone without symptomatic heart disease is not an emergency. However, your condition could be different, so ask your doctor whether there is any case in which palpitations would require further attention.

Coronary artery disease: Like any other organ in the body, the heart needs to receive blood and have a way to dispense of waste products, so there are arteries, veins, and capillaries to provide fuel to the heart and remove waste. If these arteries become narrowed or blocked, then heart damage results because the heart is not receiving enough blood. Coronary disease is worsened by high blood pressure, high cholesterol, smoking, obesity, lack of exercise and diabetes. Late in the disease, angina (chest pain) or an abnormality in the heart rhythm (arrhythmias) may be warning symptoms. Unfortunately, cardiac arrest (sudden death) may also occur.

Heart failure (acute or chronic, also known as cardiomyopathy): This term is misleading—when you hear it, you can't help but think that the heart has fully given out. Probably a better term would be "heart insufficiency," since in fact the heart hasn't "failed," but it's having a rough time. Its pumping action is deteriorating, which usually leads to an accumulation of fluid in the lungs, abdomen or legs; however there is still time for treatment. The most common cause of heart failure is a heart attack—within 6 years of a heart attack, 22 percent of men and 46 percent of women will be disabled from heart failure. Unfortunately, without aggressive treatment, heart failure symptoms worsen, and patients can die within only a few years. Anyone with a first-degree relative affected by heart failure should undergo an echocardiogram as a screening test.

Hypertrophic cardiomyopathy: This is a condition in which the heart muscle is abnormally thickened due to something other than high blood pressure. If you have hypertrophic cardiomyopathy, this plan is not intended for you unless your condition has progressed to advanced, dilated, nonobstructive cardiomyopathy. This is a type of heart disease that can be very dangerous and can be genetic. If you have it, you need to see a specialist—and also make sure your family members all get echocardiograms to make certain they are not affected. Anyone with a first-degree relative affected by hypertrophic cardiomyopathy should undergo an echocardiogram as a screening test.

Hypertension: This is the term used for persistent high blood pressure that causes damage to the heart, arteries and other organs of the body. According to the traditional definitions of hypertension, about 1 in 5 adults have this condition. In fact, it is closer to half or more. If left untreated, hypertension leads to an increased risk of heart attacks, strokes and premature death. In general, a person is considered to have hypertension when his or her blood pressure is persistently higher than 140/90, even at rest. A new designation of prehypertension refers to people with a blood pressure between 115/75 and 140/90—a group at higher risk than those with normal blood pressure. Hypertension does not cause symptoms, so is frequently referred to as a "silent killer" because individuals may have a fatal stroke or heart attack without warning. African Americans have a greater tendency to have hypertension, as do men, as well as men and women who are over-weight or drink a lot of alcohol. The fact that arteries become stiffer with age also means that older people are more likely than younger people to have high blood pressure. Even if you don't have high blood pressure by the time you reach 50, you still have a 90 percent chance of developing the problem.

Myocardial infarction: This is a medical term for a heart attack or a "coronary." A heart attack is almost always caused by the narrowing of the coronary arteries that supply the heart muscle with freshly oxy-genated blood. In contrast to the plaques that block blood flow in a patient with angina (chest pain during exertion), the blockages that cause heart attacks block the blood flow abruptly. This occurs when the fibrous covering of a relatively small but cholesterol-filled plaque ruptures. Symptoms of myocardial infarction generally develop sud-denly and may include severe, crushing pain at the center of the chest, and this pain can radiate up to the neck and out into the arms, par-ticularly the left arm. A person may also feel sweaty, short of breath, nauseated or anxious.

Valvular heart disease: This describes any type of disease that affects the heart's four valves. This occurs when the valve narrows or leaks, producing a heart murmur audible in a physical examination. While some murmurs are innocuous, others may require open-heart surgery.

If you are ever told you have a murmur, ask your doctor for an echocardiogram. This will tell you whether you need to worry; whether you need further treatment, including the need to take antibiotics to prevent an infection on the valve.

White coat hypertension: Some people have a significant increase in blood pressure when it is measured by the doctor. The pressure can be 20 or 30 points higher when measured by a doctor wearing a white coat, but normal at other times. Recent studies show that people whose blood pressure rises in the doctor's office also rises whenever they are faced with any stressful situation. Although considered to be a minimal concern by many, white coat hypertension can damage the heart and increase your risk, so it should be treated.

For more information about the symptoms of a heart attack and what to do if you think you may be having one, review Appendix A.

CHAPTER 3

Feel Better and Live Longer: The Program and How It Works

IF YOU ARE AT RISK OF CARDIOVASCULAR DISEASE, AND MOST adults are, the most powerful way to feel better and live longer is through the medicines in this plan. Recent studies show that this plan can add an average of over 10 years of life free from heart attacks or strokes for a typical 50- or 60-year-old American adult while cutting your risk of dying in half. No lifestyle program can make that claim.

The program rests on established testing strategies and treatments. The medicines are not new, but rather have been used by millions of people over decades and have been proven safe and effective.

Hundreds of medical therapies seem logical and safe when first proposed, but eventually we learn that most are dangerous, so they never make it to your pharmacy. The only way to learn whether to use them is through scientific studies that measure the effects very carefully. Testing medicines in sick people identifies even minor problems quickly, since people who are the sickest are also more sensitive to even minor side effects. Testing medicines in healthier people in studies lasting for several years allows detection of side effects caused by long-term use. Once a medicine is on the market, millions more take the medicine, which provides another opportunity to learn about its safety. All of the medicines in this program are proven safe in each of these types of scientific studies and over decades of clinical use. They are safer than many medicines and vitamins you may take without pause. In Chapter 4, you will find the data that prove how safe these medicines are.

Your Testing Plan

A crucial difference between this program and general medical practice is in the *interpretation* of the test results. Appendix B explains the way that normal ranges for tests are derived, and how these ranges that are printed on test reports can be misleading.

Here is the list of tests to determine the kinds of treatment you may need. Although it may look like quite a few tests, many are tests that should already be routinely performed, and all the blood tests can be drawn at the same time.

Blood pressure: Blood pressure should be measured in both arms at least once to be certain that the levels are equal. If they are more than 5 or 10 mm different, you should ask for a further evaluation by a cardiologist (you will probably learn that it is nothing dangerous). Thereafter, you can have the pressure measured in either arm.

Preparation for the test: none
Frequency: 20, 25 and 30 years of age and every year thereafter

Fasting cholesterol and lipid profile (blood test): The complete cholesterol profile is a must, as this includes not only the cholesterol level but also the good cholesterol (HDL), bad cholesterol (LDL) and triglyceride (this is bad, but not as bad as LDL) levels. Since the total cholesterol is (approximately) equal to the sum of HDL, LDL and triglycerides, and some types are good and some bad, you need to know the levels of the individual components. For example, if you had a very high HDL and a very low LDL, you could have an elevated total cholesterol but the lowest possible risk.

Preparation for the test: You should have this blood test after fasting for at least 8 hours in order for it to be the most accurate.
Frequency: 20 years of age and every 5 years thereafter

Diabetes screening measuring HgA$_{1c}$ and fasting blood sugar (blood test): Measuring glucose when fasting is an easy way to test for diabetes, and the HgA$_{1c}$ test provides additional information about whether you may have pre-diabetes.

Preparation for the test: after an 8-hour fast for blood sugar, but HgA$_{1c}$ can be drawn anytime

Frequency: 20 years of age and every 5 years thereafter

Electrocardiogram: This is a standard way to record the electrical activity of the heart, and it provides insight into the structure of the heart. The test is performed by placing stick-on electrodes on your chest, arms and legs to record the tiny electrical impulses your heart produces. An abnormal electrocardiogram does not mean your heart is abnormal. This test detects abnormalities pretty accurately, but it is far from perfect. When there is any suggestion of an abnormality, an echocardiogram is performed, using sound waves to take pictures of your heart.

Preparation for the test: none

Frequency: 30 years of age and every 5 years thereafter

Homocysteine (blood test): Homocysteine is a chemical that is produced in your body, and when the level is high, so is your risk of cardiovascular disease. However, there is no proof that doing anything about your homocysteine level gives you any advantage. This test is useful in understanding whether you are at higher risk than the other tests indicate, but there is nothing to do about it at this time.

Preparation for the test: none

Frequency: 40 years of age and every 5 years thereafter

CRP (blood test): The C-reactive protein (CRP) is a reflection of the inflammation in your body. If there is a lot of inflammation in the walls of your arteries, this level is higher, and if you have a cold, this level is also increased. Although a lot of things make the level go up, if there are no other apparent sources of inflammation, the CRP level correlates with your cardiovascular risk. There is no proven way to lower your risk if your level is high. Therefore, like homocysteine, this test is useful to estimate your risk of problems.

Preparation for the test: none
Frequency: 40 years of age and every 5 years thereafter

Echocardiogram (noninvasive ultrasound test): This is a way to take pictures of your heart and measure how well it is functioning. Echocardiograms are also useful in understanding the reason for heart murmurs. To get this test, you will need to be seen by a cardiologist or radiologist, although usually a trained technician performs the test, not the doctor. There is no risk with this test, and the results should be available by the next day. Doctors do not routinely perform this test unless there is a heart murmur or symptoms suggesting cardiovascular disease, but the test is a useful screening tool for heart disease for people who are middle-aged.

Preparation for the test: none
Frequency: 50 years of age and every 10 years thereafter

BNP (blood test): The level of brain naturetic peptide in your blood is a reflection of the pressure inside your heart. If your heart becomes stiff and thickened from years of high blood pressure, or weak after a heart attack or developing heart failure, the pressures rise and so does the BNP level. Many physicians advocate using this test to screen for people with structural changes in their hearts.

Preparation for the test: none
Frequency: 50 years of age and every 5 years thereafter

Additional testing: If you notice a change in your exercise capacity, whether or not the change is associated with chest pain or shortness of breath, get an echocardiogram (noninvasive ultrasound test) and possibly a stress test, if your doctor decides you need one to establish whether you have significant coronary artery disease.

Each of these tests is necessary, either to diagnose a problem or to measure more precisely your risk. None of the tests put you in danger.

If you request a test of your doctor and are told it's not necessary, be direct. Just tell your doctor you want these tests since they can tell you whether you are at risk of a heart attack, stroke or premature death. You will receive the tests. Doctors shouldn't argue with patients—

especially in a case like this, in which your concerns are reasonable. Your insurance is likely to pay for all of them (Appendix C), except for the CAT scan I discussed in Chapter 2, usually called an EBCT or ultrafast CT. This test can detect the calcium that is deposited in your arteries within the plaques that have already had small ruptures, generally ruptures that were so small that you didn't feel a thing. As I described earlier, if you have a lot of calcium deposits in your coronary arteries, you have very advanced disease and your risk of suffering a heart attack is very high. However, if your score is low, you may still be at risk, since the plaques that are the most dangerous are those without calcium that cannot be detected by this CAT scan. I do not recommend this as a standard test, although it is useful as a means to convince someone who is resisting treatment that they are at very high risk.

Strive for Optimal Health

If you don't know whether you have high blood pressure, elevated cholesterol levels, diabetes or other cardiovascular problems, the results of these tests will help you and your doctor figure it out. Then you should read the chapters in Part 3 with the steps you will need to take. Understanding the ways in which tests are interpreted before you hear your doctor's explanation will prepare you to discuss the results constructively, enabling you to control your care.

Interpretation of the Results: Optimal Health through Optimal Targets

Having results as listed below indicates you are at minimum risk.

- Cholesterol: total cholesterol < 160, LDL < 100 (or < 80 in higher risk people), HDL > 40 (men) or > 50 (women)
- Blood pressure: < 115/75
- Diabetes: Fasting blood sugar < 100, HgA_{1c} < 6%
- Electrocardiogram (ECG, EKG): normal rhythm, no evidence of hypertrophy or "nonspecific changes"

- Homocysteine: < 10 (or < 5 in higher risk people)
- CRP: < 1.0
- Echocardiogram: No evidence of enlargement of any chamber or thickening of any chamber wall
- BNP: < 100
- Stress test: No evidence of abnormal cardiovascular function with a maximal effort; ability to exercise an appropriate amount during the test

In some cases, the results of a test may lead to additional tests. For example, if the electrocardiogram shows an abnormality, undergoing an echocardiogram, and perhaps a stress test, can tell whether this abnormality is a genuine concern or not. In some cases, the information may even lead to invasive tests, such as a cardiac catheterization. Such a step is a bit scary, but here, too, you need to weigh the risks of doing the test relative to the risks of not knowing the extent of your problem.

While it is tempting not to push for further testing, that isn't always the safest approach. For example, if you were to have dangerous coronary artery disease, and the stress test does not detect it (it is only about 95 percent accurate), you and your doctor could decide not to treat. But since you actually would have a major problem that the test failed to detect, your life would be at risk. Most of the problems detected by a cardiac catheterization would respond to treatment. Because cardiac catheterization is relatively safe, although it does have its own set of risks, it can make all the difference in your treatment and your safety.

What Can You Expect?

These tests will identify treatable targets. More than half of American adults have a blood pressure above normal (greater than 115/75) and almost half have cholesterol levels that are too high (LDL greater than 100 or total cholesterol above 160).

Four types of medicines are the primary tools in the Before It Happens Plan: aspirin, statins, beta-blockers and ACE inhibitors. Each of these medicines has been used for a decade or longer by millions of people like you, each of the medicines has proven to extend life and each has a proven safety profile better than many over-the-counter medicines or vitamin supplements.

These medicines are so safe that you can consider them the equivalent of vitamins, but with proof. While few vitamins are actually proven to reduce the risk of heart disease, those with such proof are included in this plan (some appear to be dangerous and therefore are excluded). In Chapter 4, the safety of the common vitamins will be reviewed.

You can stick with this program and know that the longer you continue, the longer you stay alive.

Why Aren't All Doctors Following This Plan?

Many doctors are following this plan. I see it every day when I make rounds in the hospital. I hear about it when I talk to doctors about the way they treat themselves. But it's possible that your doctor isn't.

If not, one reason may be that your doctor is working so hard to follow the government guidelines that define the best care, that he or she is not considering your needs as an individual. It's not your doctor's fault; following those guidelines becomes second nature when you continuously hear that the best doctors strictly adhere to them. (This is the message one hears throughout four years of medical school, three to six more of training afterwards and then at every scientific meeting that follows.) The most recent guidelines for cholesterol management are known by the abbreviation NCEP/ATP-3. The National Cholesterol Education Program, Adult Treatment Panel, 3rd version, freely admits where its priorities lie. In the 372-page document, no questions are raised about the effectiveness or safety of statins, only the cost-effectiveness. Quite clearly, cost is what prevents them from recommending that you take a statin early in the development of atherosclerosis (the process of plaques forming in the walls of the arteries). The document summarizes the data that support widespread clinical use of statins, not only after a heart attack or stroke, but before suffering either one, because the efficacy (effectiveness) and safety of statins are proven.

Your doctor may not realize that those guidelines define the best care based on society's needs, not yours. As I reviewed in the prior chapters, the benefits to the individual are balanced against the cost to society. When the cost is too high, you lose.

According to ATP-3, if you have a 1 in 200 chance of having a heart attack or dying from cardiac disease in the next year, you should not be treated with a statin, even though it could reduce your risk by 25 to 50 percent. The guidelines recommend an LDL of under 130 as good enough for most of us, based on a formal analysis of the cost to society relative to the benefit of more aggressive treatment. The safety of statins is not questioned, only the cost. According to ATP-3, at today's retail prices for statins, it's too expensive to reduce your LDL to under 100, even though that would lower your risk of heart attacks, strokes and premature deaths. The guidelines calculate that a statin needs to cost under $500 per year in order to be a worthwhile investment. It's getting close. Low-dose generic lovastatin can cost as little as $430 per year, while the higher doses usually required cost a little

---

If you are a 47-year-old man with a total cholesterol of 220, LDL of 120 and HDL of 41, you have a 1 in 200 chance of having a heart attack in the next year. A statin would reduce your risk to 1 in 1,000. Your risk would be 80 percent lower. The traditional guidelines do not recommend a statin, leaving your risk 5 times higher than it could be.

If you were a 56-year-old woman with a cholesterol of 246, an HDL of 48 and an LDL of 172, you would have a 1 in 250 chance of suffering a heart attack or dying from cardiovascular disease within the next year. Reduction of your cholesterol to the targets of this plan would reduce your risk by 75 percent, to 1 in 1,000. The standard guidelines do not recommend a statin, leaving your risk 4 times higher than it could be.

more than $500 per year. Name brand fluvastatin costs only $610. The most potent statins, and those with the most overwhelming data supporting their use, are more expensive, but even so, this is not how your medical care should be determined. Instead, the target for cholesterol lowering should be based on your risk and the safety of the medications. The guidelines make their case for the current treatment targets based on financial limitations, not your personal risk. The results of your blood cholesterol test must be interpreted according to the goal of optimizing your health and minimizing your risk. Instead, this type of financial bias results in targets for treatment that effectively mean that less than optimal health is good enough.

The guidelines do not recommend treatments to minimize *your* risk, but to maximize the ratio of the benefit to society relative to the total cost to society.

Another reason you are not treated optimally by your doctor is due to other patients in his or her practice. Most people don't like to take medicines, and doctors get tired of being salespeople, trying to convince patients why they should take a pill. By this point, you should be more open to the idea of taking these medicines. But if you aren't, despite their proven safety and ability to lower your risk, you'll be willing by the time you finish the first four chapters and an applicable profile in Part 3.

Ultimately, your treatment will be optimal only if you are committed to making it so. Think back to when you were in school (or if that is too long ago, think about your approach with your children). Did you start each semester hoping for Cs? I bet you wanted As. You may have known that you were not going to get A's in certain classes, but I am sure you started each class with a strategy to achieve it if at all possible. Don't fall in the trap of accepting average health, the equivalent of getting a C for your health grade. You deserve an A.

The risk of a heart attack within a year for an average middle-aged man is 1 in 200, and of dying within the following year 1 in 800. His lifetime risk of dying in a car crash is 1 in 5,000, more than 6 times lower. You wear seatbelts and are comforted by having air bags, but where do you think you should spend the most energy?

CHAPTER 4

The Tools of the Program: Aspirin, Statins, Beta-Blockers and ACE Inhibitors

"Take two aspirin and call me in the morning."
ANONYMOUS

DOCTORS AGREE WITH THE MEDICINES IN THIS PROGRAM. I've asked. The typical exchange goes something like this:

Q: How's your cholesterol?
A: My LDL is 75 on my statin.
Q: How's your blood pressure?
A: Great on my ACE inhibitor (or beta-blocker or diuretic).
Q: Taking any other medicines?
A: Besides an aspirin?

You are likely to be a candidate for one or more of the four medicines upon which this plan is based: aspirin, statins, beta-blockers and ACE inhibitors. (The specific names of these medicines are listed in Appendix D.)

Yes, I want you to take prescription medicines. Most people pick up bottles of vitamins at the drugstore or the health food store and take vitamin C, vitamin E and a host of other vitamin and mineral supplements based on the latest magazine article they've just read. Yet when it comes to taking a prescription medicine, they hesitate, asking, "Do I really need it?"

I don't blame you for wanting an explanation. What's ironic is America's embrace of dietary supplements—to the tune of taking several billion dollars' worth! These over-the-counter vitamins and minerals have never been tested at any dose—let alone at the high dosages that are sometimes recommended by nonmedical people writing for consumer magazines. Just because they are sold over the counter doesn't mean they are risk free. Prescription medicines have the advantage of having been tested on a broad population over a long period of time, and it is unusual for the medical community to be caught by surprise with an unsafe prescription medicine.

Though not all pharmacies distribute them, every prescription has the equivalent of a "product insert"—one of those folded-up pieces of paper with teeny-tiny writing on it. If you were to take the time to decipher the information, you would be given a capsulized version of volumes of information known about the drug from studies on thousands of patients—its side effects, the medicines with which it shouldn't be combined, any contraindications of taking it, its exact contents, etc. All this has to be carefully diagnosed, tested and explained.

I'm going to step forward and offer you a complete explanation of the medicines I'm recommending because every person deserves it. If you've been taking a self-prescribed regimen of vitamins, you may be tempted to switch. The medicines in this plan save lives and do so more safely than many vitamins or over-the-counter treatments.

How Can You Tell a Medicine Is Safe?

I use a conservative approach when deciding whether to prescribe a medicine. I look for evidence that it is better than one of the medicines you are already taking or that adding it to your medicines would provide even greater benefit.

New medicines may have been tested in only a few hundred or few thousand people for several months by the time they are approved. That is not enough to know if there are additional risks that could affect you. So, although it seems likely that the new medicine would help, you still would be wise to question its efficacy and safety.

Proving a medication's safety is difficult; but knowing that a medicine is proven safe is easy. When a company studies a new drug, it knows exactly what the drug does to one part of the body, but researchers can only reasonably be sure that the drug does not affect other parts of your body adversely. Although clinical trials are performed primarily to determine that a drug is safe and effective, they also provide reassurance that it does not harm your other organ systems.

Side Effects

Medicines cause side effects in a number of ways, but just a few questions need to be addressed to prove safety. First, can really sick patients safely take it? If a medicine is safe in sick people, who have major problems with even minor side effects, then it will not pose very substantial risks in the general population. Second, do more side effects show up when healthier people take the medicines over a few years? This tells whether toxic effects build up over time. Also, such studies can eliminate the possibility of problematic interactions with other medicines. Finally, are there additional side effects or risks identified once the medicine has been released to the market for four or five years? Once tens of thousands of people have taken a medicine for a few years, you know whether you need to worry or not. Any drug on the market for more than two years with sales of over $200 million has been given to a lot of people, so you can feel reassured. You can find out whether a particular drug has been used this much by looking up the manufacturer on the web.

All four of the medicines in this program are proven to be safe under all three of the above-mentioned circumstances. All four of these medicines are proven safe in a broad array of people, with a great variety of diseases and of disease severity, which means we know these are incredibly safe medicines.

Virtually all of the minor side effects of each of the medicines in this plan are completely reversible when you stop taking them. That means you have nothing to lose by giving the program a try.

If you want to see more about the medicines, I have included in this chapter tables summarizing some of the studies with each medicine. I have not included every study; there are too many. However, I have not left out any study that suggests any risk to you. The information in each is selected to help inform your doctor. I will explain the strategies to do so in Chapter 5.

What Do Doctors Think of These Medicines?

With what is known about these medicines, why don't more doctors take the next step and prescribe preventively? Because patient education is a process. In this era of managed care, doctors simply don't have the time to educate patients about preventive measures they could take that are not well covered in the popular press. In addition, some patients are reluctant to take prescription medications unless they have noticeable symptoms that will be remedied by them.

When I talk to other doctors about this program, they give me one other response. They point out that they believe that aspirin is a medicine that everyone over 50 should take (especially men; women usually have it recommended a few years later or at onset of menopause). It's in the standard guidelines, and it's safe. I agree with that view, but in fact, of the four medicines in this plan, aspirin is the one that has the greatest risks. It's an interesting process to watch a doctor weighing the evidence supporting aspirin compared to the data supporting the use of statins, beta-blockers and ACE inhibitors. Doctors don't conclude that aspirin is more dangerous than they thought, they conclude that these other medicines are far safer than previously realized, so safe that they should be used more widely. Together, these four medicines offer proven results and are extremely safe, having been taken by millions of people for years.

Aspirin

Aspirin reduce the risks from vulnerable plaques by:

- Inhibiting platelet clumping and blood clot formation
- Reducing inflammation within the plaque
- Stabilizing plaques

Aspirin has been used for over 100 years. Thousands of studies have established its safety and usefulness. Historically, it was used to treat rheumatologic and inflammatory conditions, meaning that it treated everything from aches and pains to colds and serious infections. However, the greatest benefit of aspirin is to reduce death and disability from cardiovascular disease. Aspirin prevents heart attacks and strokes, and saves lives for those unfortunate enough to suffer one.

Aspirin works by blocking the function of platelets, the cells that form blood clots. Without aspirin, plaques that erode or rupture in your arteries will attract platelets and immune cells, triggering the formation of blood clots to seal up those erosions and ruptures. These clots can get so big that they block any blood from flowing through the artery. In a coronary artery, this leads to a heart attack or sudden death, while in an artery leading to the brain, a stroke is the result.

Taking aspirin daily can prevent blood clots from forming, thus preventing a heart attack and reducing the risk of sudden death.

Reducing Your Risk

In 1998, the FDA reviewed all the studies of aspirin's use for cardiovascular disease, with a focus primarily on the large-scale trials with a total of over 60,000 patients studied up to 7 years. They concluded that aspirin reduced the risk of heart attacks, sudden death, or coronary artery disease–related deaths.

Table 4.1   The major, randomized, controlled studies of aspirin for cardiovascular disease

Study	Dose (mg each day)	Number Studied	Description of People Studied	Result of Treatment with Aspirin
Physicians' Health Study	162.5	22,071	Healthy male doctors	Lower risk of heart attacks, lower combined risk of heart attack, stroke or cardiovascular death
British Doctors Study	500	5,139	Healthy male doctors	No benefit for heart attack risk, aspirin caused more strokes
HOT	75	18,790	High blood pressure	Lower risk of heart attack, lower risk of cardiovascular death, higher risk of stroke when blood pressure higher than 180/100 (or even close to that level)
ISIS-2	160	17,187	Heart attack	Lower risk of death
SAPAT	75	2,035	Chronic stable angina	Lower risk of heart attack and sudden death, lower risk of cardiovascular death
SALT	75	1,360	People with warning signs of stroke	Lower risk of stroke
UK-TIA	300 or 1200	2,435	People with warning signs of stroke	Lower risk of stroke, lower risk of stroke or death, more side effects with higher dose

The United States Preventative Services Task Force agreed, specifically emphasizing that the major benefit of aspirin is proven in people with at least a 4 percent risk of a heart attack within 10 years, based on the balance between aspirin's benefit and its established risk of bleeding.

The studies that the FDA reviewed included people at risk of a heart attack or stroke, and are summarized in Table 4.1.

Dosage

If one aspirin is good, two or three or four must be better, right?

Actually, no. Increasing the dosage increases the side effects without increasing the efficacy of the treatment. Because of all of the data that suggest that lower risks are associated with lower doses, I favor use of the lowest dose of aspirin that has been shown to be effective in any study, which is 81 mg once daily (equivalent to a baby aspirin). The advice to "take two aspirin, and call me in the morning" is not the best advice. "Take a baby aspirin a day, and avoid the need to call 9-1-1" is the best advice based on the data.

Safety

Low-dose aspirin is beneficial for the average American adult and reduces the risk of a heart attack by 25 percent. Balancing this benefit against the risk of bleeding means that once your yearly risk of a heart attack, stroke, or cardiovascular death is 0.4 percent or more, the advantages of taking low-dose aspirin daily (81 mg) outweigh its risks.

Aspirin is an over-the-counter medicine because of its low risk. However, aspirin should not be taken reflexively without discussing its use with your doctor, since certain medical conditions, including high blood pressure, an abnormal bleeding system and stomach disorders, could make it a riskier medicine for you. Because aspirin prevents the normal formation of blood clots, it can increase the risk of bleeding. This risk becomes a genuine concern in people with poorly controlled blood pressure and when higher doses are used.

People taking higher doses (1,200 to 1,500 mg a day, the equivalent of 4 to 5 aspirin tablets each day) are more likely to experience stomach problems, such as an upset stomach or intestinal bleeding.

Your doctor may believe that aspirin's risk is too high if you have high blood pressure, but this may not be true. As long as your blood pressure is less than 140/90, the benefits of aspirin are proven (at doses of 81 mg a day). If your blood pressure is higher, you may still benefit, but it would depend on your particular medical condition, especially your risk of a heart attack.

I do not recommend aspirin as widely as I do the other medicines in this program, based on the associated risk of bleeding, but instead recommend it for those whose benefits clearly outweigh the risk of bleeding. This distinction is important, since your risks from statins, beta-blockers and ACE inhibitors are mostly limited to reversible side effects that are at worst bothersome, but not dangerous. (Of course, you could have an unknown allergy to any medicine, but this risk is lower than your risk of not taking the medicine in almost every case.)

To understand the approach used to decide whether aspirin is right for you, consider the impact, both positive and negative, of taking aspirin as an ongoing treatment. If 1,000 middle-aged people took an aspirin daily for 5 years, 2 to 4 of them are likely to experience a significant gastrointestinal bleed, which can be serious enough to require hospitalization, blood transfusion and even in rare cases emergent procedures, especially endoscopies. In addition, up to 2 of the 1,000 could have a disabling hemorrhagic stroke.

That means that up to 6 per 1,000 middle-aged people could have a serious problem from taking aspirin daily. If you compare the safety of aspirin to the other medicines in this plan, you will see that aspirin is the one with the highest risk of all. The risks of such serious adverse effects with statins, beta-blockers and ACE inhibitors are markedly lower. Therefore, if your doctor recommends aspirin, then you know the others are safe enough for you to take as well.

The next step is to consider whether your risk of a heart attack is more than 0.4 percent each year, justifying the use of aspirin. If you are a 45-year-old man with a cholesterol level of 219, HDL of 42 and LDL of 135 with a blood pressure of 135/82, you would have a 1 in 125 chance of suffering any significant coronary event over the next year. You should receive ongoing aspirin therapy. If you are a 56-year-

---

Can I take Tylenol instead?

No, Tylenol (acetaminophen) is useful for pain, but has no benefit at all for the prevention or treatment of cardiovascular disease.

old woman with a history of hypertension, who was treated to standard goals at 132/80 but has a cholesterol level of 220, HDL of 44, and LDL of 135, you have a 1 in 200 risk of a heart attack over the next year. You should receive chronic aspirin therapy.

Most people don't think twice about the safety of aspirin, and most don't even consider it a drug. In fact, aspirin is very safe; that's why it is available without a prescription. But of the medicines in the plan, aspirin is the most dangerous one. This gives you a sense of the safety of these medicines.

Statins

Statins reduce the risks of vulnerable plaques by:

- Reducing cholesterol deposits into your arteries
- Strengthening the lining of tissue over the plaque
- Inhibiting platelet clumping and blood clot formation
- Reducing inflammation within the plaque
- Improving local control of blood flow by your arteries

Statins are used to lower cholesterol and your risk of heart attacks, strokes and death, and are the most commonly prescribed class of medicine in the world. With over 20 years of investigation and clinical use, statins have an ideal safety profile, making them one of the safest and most powerful tools to prevent death and disability.

By the mid-1970s, the medical community clearly understood that the level of cholesterol in the blood was a strong predictor of risk of heart attacks, strokes or dying from cardiovascular disease. Around this time several medications had been identified to lower cholesterol, but these drugs, which were not statins, were never widely prescribed because they were relatively difficult for patients to tolerate, causing abdominal bloating, diarrhea and hot flashes.

By the early 1980s, clinical testing began with the first statin (lovastatin). By blocking a liver enzyme called HMG CoA reductase, cholesterol synthesis was markedly reduced. Since the liver makes at least three times as much cholesterol as we eat in a typical diet, marked reduction in cholesterol levels were expected and seen.

Early studies showed only a modest effect on the size of the fatty plaques but a marked reduction in risk. The marked impact is more than can be expected based only on plaque size, and we have learned that there are many additional mechanisms whereby statins reduce clinical risk.

Reducing Your Risk

Statins are proven effective in reducing cholesterol levels, but more importantly in keeping you alive and healthy, whether you are at risk of a heart attack or have already had one. That means that well over half of all American adults could benefit from taking a statin routinely. Studies prove that statins save lives and reduce heart attacks and strokes (see Table 4.2).

While each of these studies is notable for establishing the importance of statin therapy, a few deserve special attention, including the Heart Protection Study, which reported its results in late 2001. The goal of this study was to determine whether a statin could save lives of people who appeared to be adequately treated based on standard guidelines for cholesterol management. Specifically, these patients had relatively low cholesterol levels but either had diabetes or extensive disease of their blood vessels, enough so that they had symptoms or had been hospitalized previously.

The study showed that a dose of 40 mg of simvastatin taken nightly reduced the risk of a heart attack, stroke or cardiovascular death by 24 percent, and even did so in those people whose LDL was the lowest (under 116) even before starting in the study. Based on this study, taking a statin postpones a heart attack, stroke or cardiovascular death by over 3 years even if you already have diabetes or advanced vascular disease.

Table 4.2   The major, randomized, controlled studies of statins for cardiovascular disease

Study	Statin	Dose (mg each night)	Number Studied	Description of People Studied	Result of Treatment with the Statin
4S	simvastatin	40	4,444	People with high cholesterol after a heart attack	Lower risk of death and fewer heart attacks
WOSCOPS	pravastatin	40	6,595	People 45–64 yrs old with high cholesterol	Lower risk of death and fewer heart attacks
CARE	pravastatin	40	4,159	People with cholesterol < 240 after a heart attack	Lower risk of fatal and nonfatal heart attacks, fewer strokes
AFCAPS/ TexCAPS	lovastatin	40	6,605	People with average cholesterol	Lower risk of heart attacks
LIPID	pravastatin	40	9,014	People with high cholesterol after a heart attack or with chest pains	Lower risk of death
LIPS	fluvastatin	80	1,677	People with chest pain undergoing angioplasty	Lower risk of heart attacks; fewer procedures needed
MIRACL	atorvastatin	80	3,086	People admitted to the hospital with a new heart attack or unstable chest pain	Less chest pain; tendency to reduce stroke risk
AVERT	atorvastatin	80	341	People with chest pains referred for angioplasty (half got angioplasty, the other half atorvastatin)	Less chest pain; less procedures needed
HPS	simvastatin	40	20,536	Diabetics and those with vascular disease	Lower risk of death (even in those with LDL < 116 and total cholesterol < 193 before treatment)
ASCOT	atorvastatin	10	10,305	People with high blood pressure and cholesterol under 250	Lower risk of fatal and nonfatal heart attacks
CARDS	atorvastatin	10	2,838	Diabetics with LDL under 160	Lower risk of heart attacks and strokes

Two subsequent studies evaluated whether statins could prevent heart attacks and save lives for people with high blood pressure and those with diabetes. The Anglo-Scandinavian Cardiac Outcomes Trial studied the effects of 10 mg of atorvastatin in people being treated for high blood pressure whose cholesterol levels were less than 250. (The average level for total cholesterol was 212, LDL cholesterol 133, and HDL cholesterol 51.) Those people treated with atorvastatin had their

LDL reduced to 85 and had their risk of heart attacks (fatal and nonfatal) reduced by 37 percent and their risk of strokes cut 27 percent. Similarly, the Collaborative Atorvastatin Diabetes Study showed that atorvastatin markedly reduced risk in diabetics, most of whom had coexistent high blood pressure, without any symptoms of heart disease.

In Chapter 2, I told you about two different types of plaques that develop in your arteries. The more dangerous type is the smaller, fat-filled plaques vulnerable to rupturing and causing a heart attack or worse. This is the kind that statins and the other medicines in this plan address very potently.

The other type, easier to detect, is the type that causes symptoms, but generally does not cause as many heart attacks. When a plaque of this type exists, it clogs the arteries of your heart enough to cause angina. These plaques are treated quite effectively by angioplasty (the procedure in which catheters are inserted into the arteries of your heart and the blockage is opened using stents). Statins can help with these kinds of blockages also. In 2001, a study was published called AVERT. In this study, people who were about to have an elective angioplasty were randomly treated with high doses of the statin atorvastatin, or underwent the angioplasty. Atorvastatin did a better job of reducing angina symptoms and avoiding more procedures. (If you are recommended to have an angioplasty, don't refuse just because of this study. Ask your doctor whether studies show that you need the angioplasty or why it could be better than medicines alone based on your condition. As an example, angioplasty can save your life if you are in the midst of a heart attack, but in such a situation, you would benefit from a statin in addition.)

If your LDL is very high, you start off with a bigger chance of a heart attack or dying, but you get the biggest reduction in risk by taking a statin. However, even if your cholesterol level is only slightly elevated (above 100), taking a statin reduces your relative risk by 20 to 30 percent.

Most of the investigations using statins have focused on the risks of heart attacks and premature death. Statins are proven to reduce the risk of strokes as well in several studies (see Figure 4.1).

Statins Reduce the Risk of Stroke

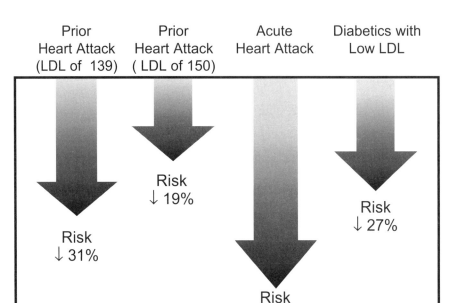

Prior Heart Attack (LDL of 139)	Prior Heart Attack (LDL of 150)	Acute Heart Attack	Diabetics with Low LDL

Risk ↓ 19%

Risk ↓ 31%

Risk ↓ 27%

Risk ↓ 50%

Figure 4.1 Most doctors talk about your risk of having a heart attack, but the risk of stroke is a big problem as well. As exemplified by these four studies, in a variety of patient types, statins reduce stroke risk by a meaningful amount.

These data are from the CARE, LIPID, MIRACL and HPS studies, respectively.

The biggest question that remains unanswered by science is how to know whether you are taking a high enough dose of statin. Recent studies report marked benefit when statins are used to lower LDL cholesterol under 80. Ongoing studies will tell us exactly how much further we should lower cholesterol, but most cardiologists I know are happiest when their patients have an LDL under 80 (and that seems to be their personal target as well). This perspective is based on several smaller studies in combination with the analysis from the Heart

Protection Study that showed impressive benefits in patients whose LDL, on average, was reduced under 80.

If you wonder whether it is worth reducing your LDL, consider the results of the Atherosclerosis Risk in the Communities Study (ARIC). When most people talk about the results of ARIC, they point out that men and women who have the highest levels of LDL are at the greatest risk of developing coronary heart disease, based on comparison of people with the highest levels (top 20 percent) compared with those with the lowest (bottom 20 percent). As you can see in Figure 4.2, the risk rises as soon as the level of LDL is above 100.

Selection and Dosage

While the statins lovastatin, simvastatin, pravastatin, atorvastatin and fluvastatin have all been studied extensively, and each reduces risk, there are differences. Simvastatin and atorvastatin are the most potent at lowering cholesterol. Simvastatin, pravastatin and atorvastatin have been studied most extensively in the large-scale randomized trials (and have proven to prevent heart attacks and strokes and to keep people alive), but lovastatin has also produced impressive benefits (and is available as a generic form). Atorvastatin and simvastatin are most commonly prescribed, and have been used for years in millions of people. For each agent, your doctor will start at a low dose and gradually increase as is necessary, based on your blood cholesterol profile.

In 2003, a new statin was released onto the market: rosuvastatin. Consistent with the approach I take in my practice, I will probably not write many prescriptions for this medicine for the first year or two it is on the market. Some of the early studies hint at possible risks at higher doses and this needs to be evaluated further. By 2005, a combination of a statin and a new agent (ezetimibe) will likely have been used enough to know that long-term safety and effectiveness match the potent effects on blood cholesterol levels. Then that combination could be considered. As with rosuvastatin, I will wait before widely recommending this combination.

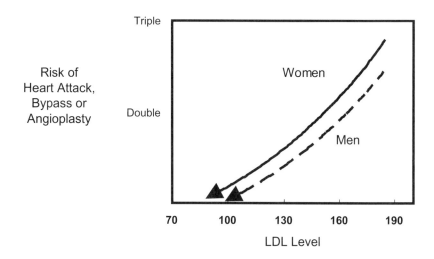

Your Risk Is Lowest
When Your LDL Is Under 100

Figure 4.2. Doctors talk as though there is something magical about reaching certain values on a test. Lowering LDL cholesterol under 160 for an asymptomatic reasonably healthy middle aged man (dotted line) or woman (solid line) is enough, according to the guidelines. But this goal is arbitrarily chosen, and in fact is purposefully chosen a bit high. If everyone in the country lowered their LDL below 160, there would be a lot less suffering in the world, and that would be much cheaper than getting everyone in the world under 130, and certainly getting everyone under 100 would be incredibly expensive.

But studies like this one, the Atherosclerosis Risk in the Communities Study (ARIC), show how much of a difference it could make to you if your LDL were much lower. Compared to an optimal goal for LDL of 100, an LDL of 130 is almost 50 percent higher risk, and an LDL of 160 is twice the risk, whether you are a man or a woman. (See Figure 8.3.)

In all the studies performed to date, as the LDL goes lower, so does your risk.

Safety

Doctors may be hesitant to prescribe statins because of the *perception* that the two main side effects could cause serious problems (irritation of the liver or muscles). All of the statins currently available in the

United States have been studied in large clinical trials. (Rosuvastatin has been used in large clinical trials, but does not yet have widespread and long-term clinical use, so I consider it separately from other statins—for now.) People studied were sick in some studies and relatively healthy in others. In all these trials, the risk of liver and muscle problems was about the same for the people getting the statin as for those getting a placebo. Statistically, it is difficult to tell if there is any difference between the risk of a statin and a placebo. The following chart shows how often the side effects occurred during a study of over 20,000 people taking a statin or a placebo for over four years in a study called the Heart Protection Study. As you can see, those taking the placebo were about as likely to have side effects as those taking the statin:

	Simvastatin	Placebo
Liver irritation		
Mild	1.3%	1.3%
Moderate	0.4%	0.3%
Muscle irritation		
Mild	0.2%	0.1%
Moderate	0.1%	0.1%
Muscle damage		
Mild	0.05%	0.01%
Severe	0.05%	0.03%

Based on data such as these and statements made by the FDA during public hearings, statins may be the safest class of prescription medications on the market. When reviewing the risk of liver failure, the most feared side effect of statins, the FDA reported that statins are safer than even the Motrin or Advil you may be taking for headaches or aches and pains. In fact, Britain's Department of Health announced in the spring of 2003 their intention to switch statins to over-the-counter status (available without a prescription) within a year. Of course there is always one exception to any rule: If you have active or chronic liver disease, you should not be taking a statin. Make sure to ask your doctor if this is relevant to you.

The most common concerns about statins are abnormalities in liver function and muscle irritation. The muscle irritation can range from a mild reaction that reveals a higher level of muscle enzymes in the blood to moderate cases where there is muscle pain or tenderness, and even to the serious medical problem of suffering muscle breakdown.

These side effects can be detected easily by a routine blood test. Standard practice is to have blood tests and doctor visits every three months and then eventually every six months. With such vigilance, any abnormalities that are detected can be easily remedied, either by reducing the dose, switching to a different statin or stopping therapy. Even given the potential for such side effects, taking a statin puts you at a lower risk than if you were to choose not to take one.

Anecdotally, I can offer you this assurance. Over the past few months, I have been asking other doctors how many times they have had a patient develop liver or muscle problems that made them stop the statin. I can't find a doctor who can remember a case. I thought I had a patient with this problem recently, but it turned out to be unrelated to his statin, and he continues to take it.

In April 1999, the FDA reviewed the safety of a broad array of medicines. Included in that analysis was a comparison of statins and specific pain medicines (those similar to Advil or Motrin) relative to the risks faced by the general population not taking either medicine. The FDA reported that the frequency of liver failure was two to four times higher in people taking these pain medicines than in the general population, while the risk for people taking statins was as low as in people not taking medicines.

Statins are the most widely prescribed class of medicines today, and the millions who take them continue to show no sign of new or unusual side effects.

Beta-Blockers

Beta-blockers protect the vasculature by:

- Reducing deposition of cholesterol within plaques
- Reducing inflammation within the plaque
- Improving local control of blood flow by your arteries
- And beta-blockers decrease the risk of sudden death, too.

Beta-blockers are standard treatment for many cardiovascular problems, most frequently for people with high blood pressure, arrythmias, a history of a heart attack (or at high risk of one) or heart failure (a weak heart).

Doctors couldn't help but be impressed with the first major study of a beta-blocker. Prior to the report in 1965 that propranolol (the first beta-blocker) reduced the risk of dying from a heart attack, there were few other treatment options available. By the 1970s, beta-blockers had also become standard tools for managing high blood pressure.

By blocking the toxic effects of adrenaline, beta-blockers prevent the arrhythmias that cause sudden death. In addition, beta-blockers protect the vasculature, independent of their ability to reduce your blood pressure.

Reducing Your Risk, Especially of Sudden Death

Many drugs can lower blood pressure or reduce symptoms of angina in people with severe coronary artery disease, but beta-blockers can do that and one more thing other drugs can't: Beta-blockers reduce your risk of sudden death.

Whatever kind of heart disease you have, sudden death is a risk; beta-blockers markedly reduce this risk (see Figure 4.3).

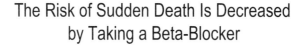

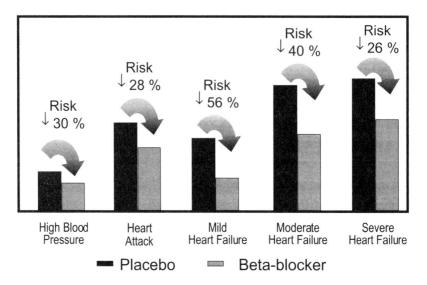

Figure 4.3 No matter what kind of heart disease you have, whether it be high blood pressure, or mild or severe heart failure, beta-blockers reduce your risk of sudden death.

Each pair of bars represents the number of people dying of sudden death whether taking a placebo (black) or a beta-blocker (gray) within a study of a particular heart condition. In all cases, the smaller gray bar means fewer people are dying of sudden death, and the amount of the difference is shown above each pair. The bars get bigger as you look from left to right because the studies towards the right include sicker people.

Selection and Dosage

One of the functions of a beta-blocker is to lower the heart rate, and in so doing it lowers blood pressure. It isn't surprising that blood pressure could go too low, but as long as your doctor starts with low doses, you shouldn't have a problem with this.

Your doctor has several options when choosing a specific beta-blocker for you and generally will make the selection based on his or her recent experience and sense of the effectiveness and tolerability of the individual drugs.

To really know which drug is best requires a study comparing the drugs against each other. That rarely happens, but it did for beta-blockers. The COMET (Carvedilol or Metoprolol European Trial) study, started in 1996, compared the beta-blockers carvedilol and metoprolol in people with heart failure and reported in mid-2003 that people taking the beta-blocker carvedilol were at significantly reduced risk of dying than those taking metoprolol. Although this study only focused on people with heart failure (a weak heart), it is persuasive evidence that all beta-blockers are not the same, and specifically that at least one deserves to be on a higher tier than other beta-blockers.

There are many studies using beta-blockers in cardiovascular disease, and I have summarized some of them in Table 4.3.

Table 4.3   The major, randomized, controlled clinical trials of beta-blockers for cardiovascular disease

Study	Beta-Blocker	Dose (mg each day)	Number Studied	Description of People Studied	Result of Treatment with the Beta-Blocker
MAPHY	metoprolol	200	3,234	High blood pressure	Lower risk of sudden death, lower risk of death from any cardiovascular cause
ISIS-1	atenolol	100	16,027	Ongoing heart attack	Lower risk of death
UKPDS	atenolol	100	1,148	Diabetic, high blood pressure	Lower risk of heart failure
Norwegian	timolol	20	1,884	Recent heart attack	Lower risk of death
BHAT	propranolol	160	3,837	Recent heart attack	Lower risk of death, lower risk of sudden death, lower risk of another heart attack
CAPRICORN	carvedilol	50	1,959	Recent heart attack and a weak heart	Lower risk of death, lower risk of another heart attack
MERIT-HF	metoprolol	200	3,991	Heart failure	Lower risk of death, lower risk of sudden death
COPERNICUS	carvedilol	50	2,289	Heart failure	Lower risk of death, lower risk of sudden death
COMET	carvedilol vs. metoprolol	50 v 100	3,029	Heart failure	Lower risk of death with carvedilol

Safety

With widespread use in virtually all cardiovascular diseases, beta-blockers are proven safe and effective. The reduction in risk of sudden death in people who have high blood pressure, a history of a heart attack or heart failure is a most compelling reason to include this agent in your regimen.

Twenty years ago beta-blockers achieved a reputation for being likely to cause fatigue, depression and impotence, but perception is frequently different from reality. Just recently a study examined whether this is true. The study showed that beta-blockers did not cause depression more than the placebo did, but were associated with more fatigue (18 patients had fatigue for each 1000 treated). People chose to continue taking the beta-blocker anyway, presumably because the fatigue was not a big deal compared to the risk of death. Impotence was infrequent (5 in 1,000 men). For those who experience impotence, the problem completely resolves after decreasing the dose or stopping the medicine.

Other than these reversible side effects, beta blockers are quite safe. This is a group of medicines that have been used for over three decades in millions of people. They are so safe that a beta-blocker is the first choice for the treatment of high blood pressure or arrhythmias in pregnancy. It won't even affect an unborn child. That is very safe.

Many doctors think they should not use a beta-blocker in diabetics. The beta-blockers that were marketed up through the 1980s worsened glucose control slightly, and theoretically could mask the symptoms associated with low blood sugar. In preliminary studies, carvedilol appears to have different effects than other beta-blockers, in that it slightly but significantly improves glucose control. Compared to the beta-blocker metoprolol, carvedilol decreases the risk of developing diabetes in people who already have cardiovascular disease (specifically, those with heart failure).

If you have severe asthma, pain in your leg muscles when walking caused by severely narrowed arteries in your legs (claudication) or a slow heart rate (especially if it is caused by "heart block"), a beta-blocker could worsen symptoms from these problems. But if you have any of these conditions, ask your doctor if you may still be able to tolerate and benefit from a beta-blocker.

ACE Inhibitors

ACE inhibitors prevent plaque rupture by:

- Enhancing strength of the cap overlying the plaque
- Reducing deposition of cholesterol within plaques
- Reducing inflammation within the plaque
- Improving local control of blood flow by your arteries

Angiotensin-converting enzyme inhibitors (ACE inhibitors) have been used for the treatment of cardiovascular disease for over 20 years. Initially used for the treatment of advanced disease (heart failure) and high blood pressure, in the past few years studies have proven even more powerful impact as treatment to prevent heart attacks, strokes, death due to cardiovascular disease and complications of diabetes. Over the past two decades, ACE inhibitors have been one of the most frequently used prescription medicines of any type for any condition.

When ACE inhibitors were first introduced in the late 1970s, the medical community was convinced that their potent benefits resulted from the relaxation of constricted blood vessels, lowering blood pressure and improving the efficiency of the heart. Already proven to lower blood pressure effectively, studies in the late 1980s proved that ACE inhibitors helped people with heart failure feel better and live longer. In the early 1990s, ACE inhibitors also proved to reduce the risk of death in people who suffered a heart attack.

ACE inhibitors reduce the production of the hormone angiotensin-2, which is intimately involved in the development and vulnerability of plaques as well as the development of hypertension. When angiotensin-2 is produced by the cells in the artery wall, the vessel constricts, leading to increases in blood pressure and lower blood flow in that region. This is a useful tool for the body, enabling ideal distribution of blood flow to the organs and muscles that need it most. Over time, as the cells in the walls of the arteries are exposed to angiotensin-2, they begin to get bigger and stronger, a process called hypertrophy. This enables them to constrict with greater responsiveness, but it also leads to stiffer arteries and increases in blood pressure even when angiotensin-2 is no longer being released.

Angiotensin-2 also stimulates cells within the plaques to grow, leading to further immune activation and instability of these plaques. Even more notable are the autopsy findings of people who die suddenly. Angiotensin-2 is formed in high amounts right at the spot of plaque rupture, along with marked activation of the immune system. Although it could be present as the result of the plaque rupture, studies show that angiotensin-2 is a major cause of the rupture.

ACE inhibitors restore normal function and improve structural changes in your blood vessels and heart. By improving the function of the cells on the vessel surface and the muscle cells underneath, as well as their interaction, ACE inhibitors restore the efficiency of local blood flow distribution. When the muscle cells are thickened, ACE inhibitors don't lower blood pressure as quickly, since they first exert a more gradual effect of regression of this muscle thickening.

ACE inhibitors reduce risks via additional mechanisms. By reducing immune activation in the walls of the arteries, inflammation and fragility of your plaques is reversed, reducing the likelihood of rupture. If an erosion or rupture of plaques does occur, and a clot begins to form, ACE inhibitors act on your blood clotting system to reduce formation of clots and prevent obstruction of blood flow within the artery. ACE inhibitors can reduce the impact of stress, even if you can't. In an animal model of psychosocial stress–induced hypertension, after several weeks of ACE inhibitor treatment, blood pressure returns toward normal.

The literature provides a very clear picture: ACE inhibitors may exert more of their beneficial clinical effects by stabilizing plaques, reducing inflammation, restoring vascular function and reducing clotting tendency than they do by reducing blood pressure, but they do that well, too.

People with diabetes or vascular disease, even without high blood pressure or heart failure, have a high risk of heart attacks or strokes. The HOPE study investigated whether the ACE inhibitor ramipril could reduce that risk, and in early 2000 reported that the ACE inhibitor prevented death and disability. Prior scientific studies suggested this would be the result, and the results were confirmed in 2003 by the study EUROPA.

Selection and Dosage

There are many choices of ACE inhibitors, and no trial proves that one is better than another. Many doctors will prescribe one for you that you only need to take once a day, for convenience. However, there are some mechanistic reasons why some ACE inhibitors could be better than others. Since angiotensin-2 is a trigger for plaque rupture, and since it is made within the tissues, not just on the surface, taking an ACE inhibitor that penetrates into the tissue would seem better. Despite this pharmacologic distinction, no study has evaluated the clinical differences between ACE inhibitors that can and cannot penetrate into the plaque, so there is no proof that this is more than a biochemical advantage.

Nonetheless, why not pick one that is "tissue avid" if there is even a slight chance it is better? Ramipril, trandolopril and perindopril are three tissue-avid agents with proven benefit in large-scale trials. Quinapril is also tissue avid, but it has not been proven to reduce the risk of heart attacks, stroke or death (it was studied primarily to show its benefit on blood pressure and quality of life). I think of a tissue-avid ACE inhibitor as an opportunity for "extra credit": It can't worsen your grade, but it could turn your B into an A.

An ACE inhibitor will keep you alive and healthy. Many studies of ACE inhibitors show their safety and effectiveness, and I have summarized several of them in Table 4.4.

Table 4.4   **The major, randomized, controlled trials of ACE inhibitors for cardiovascular disease**

Study	ACE Inhibitor	Dose (mg each day)	Number Studied	Description of People Studied	Result of Treatment with the ACE Inhibitor
SAVE	captopril	150	2,231	Recent heart attack and weak heart	Lower risk of death
TRACE	trandolapril	4	1,749	Recent heart attack and weak heart	Lower risk of death, lower risk of sudden death
AIRE	ramipril	10	2,206	Recent heart attack with heart failure	Lower risk of death
SOLVD-Prevention	enalapril	20	4,228	Weak heart but no symptoms	Lower risk of developing heart failure
SOLVD-Treatment	enalapril	20	2,569	Weak heart with heart failure	Lower risk of death
CONSENSUS	enalapril	40	253	Severe end-stage heart failure	Lower risk of death
ISIS-4	captopril	100	58,050	Ongoing heart attack	Lower risk of death
GISSI-3	lisinopril	10	19,394	Ongoing heart attack	Lower risk of death
HOPE	ramipril	10	9,297	Diabetes or vascular disease	Lower risk of death, lower risk of heart attack, lower risk of stroke
PROGRESS	perindopril	4	6,105	Recent stroke (or a warning of one)	Lower risk of stroke, lower risk of heart attack
EUROPA	perindopril	8	12,218	Coronary artery disease	Lower risk of heart attack, sudden death or any other cardiovascular cause of death

ACE inhibitors lower the risk of damage to your heart, brain and kidney; they prevent diabetes and they can save your life. But their effect is not based only on blood pressure lowering. In a study that compared an ACE inhibitor to another blood pressure medicine (called a calcium channel blocker), the two were equally effective at lowering blood pressure, but patients taking the ACE inhibitor suffered far fewer cardiovascular problems. In another study, a calcium channel blocker lowered blood pressure more than the ACE inhibitor, but the patients taking the ACE inhibitor still were less likely to suffer cardiovascular events.

The HOPE study proved how widely ACE inhibitors need to be used. If you have high blood pressure, diabetes or any evidence of vascular disease, ACE inhibitors will protect you. If your cholesterol is elevated, or if you are a smoker or are significantly overweight, you have more extensive vascular disease than normal, and ACE inhibitors will protect you, too.

Safety

There are no major toxic effects associated with ACE inhibitors, but as with all medicines, there are possible side effects. The most common risk associated with ACE inhibitor therapy is the development of a cough (it occurs in fewer than 5 percent of those who take the medication). A cough caused by the medicine is not associated with mucous production, fever, weight loss or any pain. If you are taking an ACE inhibitor and have a cough along with any of these symptoms, see your doctor promptly, as the cough is not a result of the ACE inhibitor.

If you develop a mild cough, I generally recommend continuing ACE inhibitor therapy. A medicine called an ARB (angiotensin receptor

Frequency of symptoms caused by an ACE inhibitor, leading patients to stop treatment in a large randomized trial (SAVE trial). This study covered 4.5 years of treatment.

	ACE inhibitor	Placebo
Dizziness	2.9%	2.2%
Cough	2.4%	0.8%

blocker) could be substituted, but is not proven to be quite as good as an ACE inhibitor at keeping people alive. However, if you (or your spouse) find that the cough interferes with normal functioning or sleep, taking an angiotensin receptor blocker is the second best medicine. These agents function in a similar fashion and appeared to be almost as good, but not exactly equivalent to, an ACE inhibitor. They have been used in studies with large numbers of patients over many years and have been very widely used clinically. They appear to have a favorable safety profile. However, ACE inhibitors remain the gold standard.

ACE inhibitors can sometimes interfere with kidney function. Many refer to this as the risk of renal failure, but these medicines do not cause kidney failure if you follow the advice of your doctor. The ACE inhibitor changes the way blood flows within the kidney, so that a blood test of kidney function can appear abnormal. If the change is minimal, ACE inhibitor therapy should be continued, providing the small changes do not get worse. If the change is dramatic, ACE inhibitor therapy should be stopped, with the expectation that kidney function will return to normal.

ACE inhibitors rarely cause angioedema, which you would notice as numbness and/or swelling in and around the mouth and throat. If you have these symptoms, you should stop the medicine and call your doctor. It generally goes away after stopping the medicine. In the HOPE study, this happened to 14 of 4,645 people taking ramipril and to 5 of 4,652 people taking placebo (0.3 percent and 0.1 percent, respectively). No one died from this problem and it went away after stopping the medicine. If you have experienced this problem, you shouldn't take the medicine again and you should tell any new doctor that you had this problem, since it could be worse the second time.

ACE inhibitors are potent cardiovascular medications; they can markedly change the function and the structure of the arteries in a way that reduces your risks of a heart attack, stroke or death. The mechanisms of action are broad, and complementary with the other medicines that are part of this plan.

> All risks are relative; yours is lower with these medicines than without them.

Trial	Vitamins Deaths / # Treated	Placebo Deaths / # Treated
CHAOS	36 / 1,035	26 / 967
GISSI-Prevention	487 / 5,660	527 / 5,664
HOPE	535 / 4,761	537 / 4,780
HPS	1,446 / 10,329	1,389 / 10,289
WAVE	16 / 212	6 / 211
Total	2,520 / 21,997	2,485 / 21,911
Percent Chance of Dying	11.5%	11.3%

What about Vitamins?

Vitamins, nutritional supplements and herbal remedies are sold to you without the need for any scientific proof of safety or effectiveness. Each year, billions of dollars are spent on vitamins because consumers feel they will be healthier by taking them. But this perception should be based on some scientific evidence, and the best evidence (summarized in the charts on this page and on page 64) show that a variety of vitamins either have no effect on your risks or can actually increase it. This is true for anti-oxidant vitamins, beta-carotene and vitamin E. You may feel reassured that anti-oxidant vitamins do not increase your risk of death if you have heart disease (or those at risk of developing it), but they don't reduce the risk either.

Anti-oxidant vitamins also increase your risk if you need treatment for high cholesterol. If you have coronary artery disease and abnormal cholesterol, you could be treated with a statin or the combination of a statin and anti-oxidant vitamins. A study published in the *New England Journal of Medicine* showed that the addition of anti-oxidant vitamins makes plaques get bigger instead of smaller and increases the risk of a heart attack.

The four medicines in this program are safer than taking anti-oxidant vitamins.

Some vitamins do increase your risk of dying. Doctors at the Cleveland

The risk of cardiovascular death is 10 percent higher if you take beta-carotene (Vitamin A).

Trial	# People	Beta-Carotene	Placebo
ATBC	29,133	5.3%	4.9%
CARET	18,314	2.4%	1.7%
HPS	20,536	8.6%	8.2%
NSCP	1,621	0.7%	1.5%
PHS	22,071	3.1%	2.8%
WHS	39,876	0.1%	0.1%
Total	**131,551**	**3.4%**	**3.1%**

Clinic performed an exhaustive analysis of the effects of vitamins on the risk of death, based on all studies ever published (which included over 130,000 people). People taking vitamin A (as beta-carotene, 60 to 200 mg a day) had a 7 percent overall higher risk of dying and a 10 percent higher risk of dying from cardiovascular disease. Although the size of the risk is small, these were statistically significant risks, which to you means that this risk is real and more than a mere mathematical conclusion.

One type of vitamin seems to make sense: high dose B vitamins. In your body, a chemical is produced called homocysteine, which worsens plaques in blood vessels. Your risk of heart disease is higher if you have a high homocysteine level. B vitamins can lower homocysteine levels, but the important question is whether it affects your risk.

The four medicines in this program are safer than beta-carotene.

There are only a few studies assessing the effects of B vitamins. In most cases, the studies show no effect. But when people were studied who had undergone procedures to open up blocked arteries in their hearts (angioplasty and stent implantation), one study showed that B vitamins help the angioplasty work better while another study showed the opposite. At this point in time, despite the circumstantial information, the scientific data raise the possibility that B vitamins may be dangerous, in the same way that vitamin A or anti-oxidant vitamins can be, and should not be used routinely.

If you believe that your regular vitamins are fine and the medicines recommended in the Before It Happens Plan seem dangerous, you are making the wrong assumption—one that could cost you your life.

> The four medicines in this program are safer than vitamin B supplements.

Your doctor may start you on the medicines in this program simultaneously or sequentially, depending on your medical condition. With the addition of these medicines, you will need to have follow-up visits and blood tests to make sure you are receiving the right dose to provide the maximum effectiveness with no signs of any irritation to your vital organs. To understand which of these medicines you will need, check the chapters in Part 3 that apply to you.

PART 2

How to Work with Your Doctor

CHAPTER 5

Talking with Your Doctor

START OUT WITH YOUR SIMPLE REQUEST. "I WANT TO GO ON
the Before It Happens Plan." If your doctor is familiar with my theo-
ries, you're all set. You will have the right tests and the results will lead
to a treatment plan that will minimize your risks. If your doctor
doesn't know the plan particulars, inform him or her:

- "The Before It Happens Plan advocates for the strictest possible control of blood pressure and cholesterol levels to minimize my risks of
  heart attacks, strokes or death. Based on all the studies, the plan recommends using aspirin, statins, beta-blockers and ACE inhibitors."

If your doctor doesn't recognize the plan by name or description,
you will need to explain your goals. Tell your doctor that you want to
be treated more aggressively. Acknowledge that you'll need some
tests, and explain that you would be willing to take the medicines that
will minimize your risk of suffering a heart attack or stroke, as long as
they are proven to be safe.

It shouldn't be hard; most doctors want to treat patients more
aggressively but are frustrated by patients' resistance to getting more
tests or taking more medicines. In fact, whenever a new medicine is
proven to save lives, doctors try to figure out how to convince their
patients to take it, expecting that it will be a difficult task.

Here's the plan for your conversation, with the understanding
that you may only have time to address these two points. First,
implement the testing plan. This shows how high your risk is and

identifies treatment targets. Second, let the scientific evidence dictate the optimal medicines to minimize your risk (which will include some or all of the medicines of this plan).

- "I am reading a book that says I should have my blood pressure and cholesterol checked, as well as have a specific test for diabetes, to learn if I may be at higher risk than I thought of a heart attack, stroke or even dying."

- "This book says that my risk is minimized if my blood pressure is less than 115/75 and my cholesterol is less than 160, with an LDL of under 100."

- "I know most patients don't want to hear that they need to take medicines, and neither do I, but the book says that studies prove the usefulness of aspirin, statins, beta-blockers and ACE inhibitors as especially useful to minimize my risks."

The two-point plan to discuss with your doctor:

● ●

- Get the tests to determine your risk and identify treatment targets.

- Initiate necessary medications to prevent a heart attack or stroke.

- "Am I a candidate for these medicines to reach my goals of a blood pressure under 115/75 and an LDL cholesterol of less than 100?"

If your doctor doesn't seem to understand you, visiting http://beforeithappens.com/md on the web will provide him or her with more details about the scientific basis for the plan. You can also refer your doctor to the *British Medical Journal*, which published a series of articles in their June 28, 2003 issue. Those reports describe the use of a "one-size fits all Polypill" containing the medicines in this plan plus a vitamin. (However, use of this vitamin is not based on conclusive scientific proof, as I explain in Chapter 4.) Nonetheless, the principles are similar.

The tests you need are standard, and you should get them even if you don't ask. But just to make sure, here is a conversation that a patient had with her doctor recently. You can follow the same script, and in all likelihood, the responses from your doctor will be similar.

PATIENT: "I'd like you to perform these tests on me."
DOCTOR: "You don't need them; you're fine."
PATIENT: "Is there any risk to these tests?"
DOCTOR: "No."
PATIENT: "Then what is the downside, especially if we identify something that needs treatment?"
DOCTOR: "Okay, I'll order them."

To direct the conversation, you should have your script written down. Then pick up to three graphs or tables in the book to show your doctor. You don't have to memorize everything, just read your questions off a piece of paper you bring with you (or take this book or go to my website to download information for your doctor, http://beforeithappens.com).

> Don't ask *if* you can have a few minutes, don't ask *if* your doctor has enough time to answer your list of questions. You don't want to give your doctor a chance to set limits on the discussion before you even get started. If your doctor does not have time, simply ask when he or she will be available. Your doctor needs to be willing and able to discuss important issues with you, or identify a colleague who can. If your doctor is not willing to accommodate you, it may be time for a second opinion.

Understand Your Doctor

The practice of medicine has become the business of medicine. Each year, the amount that doctors are paid for office visits and procedures decreases while the amount of paperwork increases. Most doctors compensate by seeing more patients, which makes your appointments shorter.

Knowing your doctor's personality makes a difference. Your friends and relatives have different interests, so you speak to each about different things in different ways. The same is true about doctors. Some may be delighted if you engage in a discussion about your health, while others may be less receptive at first. Consider your doctor's personality (for example, "likes the facts quickly," "wants to know how you feel," "will want to study the science behind all of it") and remember that you need to get to the point pretty quickly. You may only have 5 or 6 minutes.

However, if your doctor does not say yes immediately, then you will need to have a conversation in a way that enlightens your doctor. This is not as hard as it seems. When my daughter first went to school, I would ask her what she did. She would say, "Nothing at all," so I learned the usefulness of asking specific questions. Asking an open-ended question and hoping for an adequate response just doesn't work. If you want information, people don't just give it to you. You need to ask, and usually you need to ask progressive questions to get to the fundamental issues. You will see how such a strategy can direct your doctor to treat you optimally.

Asking "yes or no" questions doesn't work much better. Think about these questions. "Is there anything else I should know? Is there anything else I should do? Are there other tests or treatments I should consider? Is there an advantage to me seeing a specialist for a second opinion?" If you ask your doctor questions like these, the response will likely be a simple "No." How can I be so sure? If your doctor thought the answer to any of these questions were yes, he or she would have already given you the additional information. For your doctor, giving information to you only after you ask such a question would be like admitting that he or she forgot to tell you something crucial. Can you imagine your doctor saying, "Oh yes, there was one thing I forgot to tell you. It's a good thing you reminded me, because if we didn't take care of this last thing, you would likely suffer a stroke before your next appointment."

You may feel uncomfortable asking your doctor questions. Will your doctor be angry or put off? If so, you need to find out now. A doctor who can't handle questions about your risk of a heart attack or a stroke is unlikely to develop that skill later if you need it in a crisis.

If you can't get specific answers, you may need to get a second opinion to identify your next step. Many doctors will answer your questions with a combination of standard English and medical jargon, making you more uncertain. If your doctor can't answer your questions in a way you can understand fully, say so. Generally a nurse or associate can clarify the issues.

You can structure your conversations in many ways, but you should include three components. First, establish your goal: to stay healthy. Then, give your doctor a reason (or an excuse) why you have not been treated optimally, by acknowledging that most patients do not want to take medicines. This removes any blame, hopefully keeping your doctor from reacting defensively. Third, establish that you are willing to take additional medicines if they can extend your life. In this way, you lead your doctor to a decision point: Is there any reason why you shouldn't get these life-saving treatments?

Know the Roadblocks

Your doctor's schedule seems too full.

When you make the appointment, you could ask for more time than usual, but you probably won't get it. You could ask if there are certain days or times when you are likely to get a bit more time. (For example, in many offices you would want to be scheduled first, since doctors tend to fall behind schedule as the day progresses and may find themselves in a hurry to catch up.)

What if your doctor thinks your treatment is good enough?
....

Just as no one is a "little bit pregnant" you do not have cardiovascular disease that is "borderline" or "nothing to worry about."

The data in Part 3 prove that your risk is high even when your problems are borderline. This plan will minimize your risk, and the chapters in Part 3 will enable you to explain to your doctor how he or she can save your life by treating these borderline problems.

During your appointment, you need to establish quickly that you understand your doctor's time is at a premium. Asking whether your doctor can speak about your risk of a heart attack or stroke gets the dialogue started, but you also need to let your doctor know that you are willing to finish the discussion later, as long as there is a definite time established to do so.

Will there be another visit? Does your doctor want to answer the questions in a phone call, or via email? Make sure you leave the room with an understanding of how the issues can be addressed within the next couple of weeks (while the conversation is fresh in his or her mind). If you are clear with your doctor that you understand the time limitations, you are more likely to form an effective partnership.

If your doctor still does not have time, simply ask when he or she will be available "to discuss these issues of life and death." At this point, if your doctor is not accommodating, you don't have a doctor who is right for you. Your doctor needs to be willing and able to explain important issues with you, or to identify a colleague who can. If not, this may be a signal that you need a second opinion.

Your doctor is defensive.

Your doctor may respond defensively to your forwardness. This could be a sign of insecurity or perhaps unfamiliarity with the evidence. Realize that not many patients ask questions; they do what they are told.

If your doctor seems unfamiliar with the scientific evidence, let me make it easier. Tell him or her to email me and I will send lecture materials to explain the scientific basis for this plan. The email address is: sendslides@beforeithappens.com

You could also leave behind some photocopies of the charts that relate to you. Just leave them with the office staff as you leave, and let them know that your doctor will be looking for that information later.

This will give him or her the chance to review the information and present his analysis to you at the next visit.

Your doctor is not paying attention to you.

If it appears that your doctor is not concentrating on you, ask when you can schedule another appointment to finish the discussion about how he can help you reduce your risk of suffering a heart attack, stroke or premature death.

- "It seems to me that your office is even busier than usual today. Can your staff schedule another appointment for me in the next couple of weeks, so that I can learn how you can help me reduce my risk of suffering a heart attack, stroke or premature death, in addition to me working on my lifestyle?"

If your doctor responds by asking for clarification, you are ready to move forward with your prepared questions. If not, make the next appointment. Don't get angry or frustrated. Focus on improving the quality of your medical care.

Your doctor tells you his or her usual (or the standard) approach.

If possible, you don't want your doctor to tell you what he or she usually does for someone like you. You already know, since that is how your doctor already treats you, following the standard approach to medical care that is good for society but leaves you at risk. As strange as it may seem, if you make the mistake of letting your doctor say what he or she currently does, the dynamic of the process changes. Then you face the task of trying to convince your doctor to change his or her approach. Instead, feign ignorance that your doctor has not treat-ed you optimally, and let him or her follow your questions to arrive at the conclusions based on the scientific proof, ultimately leading your doctor to treat you optimally and minimizing your risk.

Perhaps your doctor's standard approach is to follow this plan, but there are reasons why you should not receive the treatment. Listen carefully to what your doctor says. He or she may be trying to assert control, and may be simply taking a circuitous route to where you want to go anyway. Let your doctor save face; don't interrupt. It may seem that he or she doesn't understand what you are asking, but it may be that your doctor's way is to act as though everything is his or her idea.

He may be explaining to you why you are not a candidate for components of this plan, but if that is the case, the message should be clear. You also should understand why you are not, and if that is not clear, ask.

- "Do you mean I am not a candidate for this plan? If not, can you explain to me why these safe medicines would not be useful to reduce my risk of a heart attack or stroke even a little bit?"

Not everyone is a candidate.

Most American adults will benefit from treatment with one or as many as all four of the medicines in this plan, but some don't need them and most don't need them all (yet). That's why the Before It Happens Plan is customized for you.

If your doctor tells you that you are not a candidate for any of the medicines in the plan, he or she should explain the reasons in a way that is clearly understandable. If not, ask for clarification, especially if your test results are above the optimum levels of the Before It Happens Plan. If there is any question in your mind that has not been completely clarified, you should get a second opinion.

A Reminder: Why This Is Your Job

Treatment guidelines take into account the scientific data in the context of standard clinical practice and the cost relative to the benefit for society. If they would consider clinical practice and experience exclusively, the guidelines could create a standard of care that would be optimal for you. But by focusing on costs, the guidelines do not address your best interests. Considering the financial impact seems necessary for the sake of society, but doctors making treatment decisions don't always seem to understand that this is the perspective of the guidelines.

There are many reasons why your doctor may recommend specific treatments other than those in this plan. The data supporting stricter control of your blood pressure and cholesterol are irrefutable; but some doctors may choose other medicines. In most cases, these alternative choices are likely to be made because of the belief that the data do not prove that treatment using ACE inhibitors and beta-blockers is better than using diuretics or calcium channel blockers. In such a case, your doctor should explain to you why a different treatment is chosen, in a way you can understand.

- "It seems we agree that I should be treated with medicines to lower my blood pressure to under 115/75 and my LDL under 100, in order to minimize my risk of heart attacks or strokes. With the safety and effectiveness of aspirin, statins, beta-blockers and ACE inhibitors so well established, why are you choosing different medicines for me?"

In contrast, if your doctor resists treating you because of a belief that the data do not support stricter targets than the guidelines recommend, or because the cost to society would be too great for you to be treated this way, you have a problem. Making decisions for your care based on the cost to society is simply unacceptable (although the cost to you is reasonable to consider). The only thing that matters is the impact on you. When I became a doctor, I vowed to protect and care for my patients. When I graduated and became a licensed physician, no one asked me to uphold any financial restraint for the benefit of the health care system. I became a doctor to treat patients. When I am a patient, I want my doctor to treat me based on my needs (maximum benefit with minimum risk), and that is how you should be treated.

Be ready to tell your doctor this, so he or she knows to consider your risks and not society's needs when making treatment decisions:

- "If a medicine is safe and decreases my risk of a heart attack or stroke by even a small amount, a few percentage points, I want that advantage."

Of course you want to reduce your risk by 50 percent or more, and that is the typical effect of this program. But every little bit of improvement is worthwhile. While many doctors don't consider a treatment worthwhile if the benefit is only a 5 or 10 percent reduction in your risk of dying, I know I would be happier if I were even 2 or 3 percent safer. You should look for any edge you can get; it is your life, after all. Your doctor should consider your risk of treating compared with not treating. If a medicine provides only a small chance of saving your life, but it is proven to be safe, it is better to take it than not to take it. As you read the chapters in Part 3 that are relevant to you, remember that the recommendations are based on your long-term safety with the medicines compared to not taking the medicines.

Booking the Appointment

Pick up the phone and make the call now. The rest of the plan is even easier to follow.

CHAPTER 6

Your Tests and Your Results

YOU NEED THREE KEY TESTS NOW: 1) MEASUREMENT OF YOUR blood pressure, 2) blood tests for cholesterol profile, and 3) blood tests for diabetes (the blood tests should be after not eating or drinking for at least 8 hours). Every doctor in the country can perform these tests, or order them quite easily at the time of your visit, and all will recognize the need to identify whether you have high blood pressure, abnormal cholesterol or diabetes. These tests will identify how to implement your personalized version of this plan immediately. All the other tests are important, but you will have time to schedule them later.

Even if your doctor is resistant to your requests to implement the plan, no doctor should tell you not to have these screening tests. These testing recommendations are not different from what your doctor should do already. Once the results are back, even a resistant doctor will want to be a good doctor. It will be straightforward to get yourself optimally treated based on the results of these tests.

Make an appointment to discuss the results of your tests, either in person or by phone. It needs to be a conversation, not just someone leaving you a message.

> **Tests You Need**
> ....
> • Blood pressure measurement
> • Cholesterol profile (blood test)
> • Diabetes screening (blood test)

Your Test Results

The test results are reported as actual numbers along with normal ranges and treatment goals. As I explained in Chapter 3, the "normal" ranges in the standard guidelines are not good enough. Further, the goals for treatment cannot be based purely on treatment guidelines, but must consider the scientific evidence.

Blood Pressure

You should have your blood pressure measured every time you visit a doctor. At least once have it measured in both arms to make sure that it doesn't matter which arm is used during subsequent visits. Some people have a 10- to 15-point difference between their arms. This usually does not mean anything is dangerous or abnormal, but it should lead to a discussion with a cardiologist.

Lowering your blood pressure below 115/75 minimizes your risk of blood pressure–related heart attacks and strokes (see Figure 6.1). That may sound strange, but there is a very specific message here. High blood pressure is one of the main causes of heart attacks and strokes, but not the only one, so lowering your blood pressure doesn't mean you don't need to work on the other causes. Two other major causes, abnormal cholesterol and diabetes, are discussed later in this chapter.

The recent guidelines accept substandard control (blood pressure of 130/80 to 140/90) and leave people at increased risk. The standard recommendation for people with diabetes is a blood pressure target of 130/80, as is the case for those with kidney dysfunction (and should be for those with heart failure). The recent guidelines acknowledge the fact that lowering blood pressure by 20 points will cut your risk in half. That means that reducing your blood pressure from a level that is good enough according to the standard goal (135/85, for example) to my stricter goal (115/75) cuts your risk in half (see Figure 6.1).

Even "borderline" blood pressure should raise concern. Many doctors believe that increases in blood pressure during office visits are not important. While it's okay to recheck it at the next visit in a month or two if it is "borderline," even these occasional increases during a doctor's visit (white coat hypertension) lead to changes in the structure of the heart and increased risk to you, risk that can be reversed following the plan in Chapter 7. (See Figure 7.2.)

Your Risk Is Minimized
When Your Blood Pressure Is Under 115/75

Risk of Death
from a Stroke
(by age)

Risk of Death
from a Heart Attack
(by age)

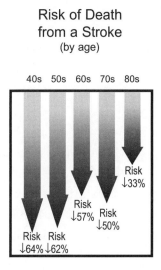
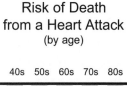
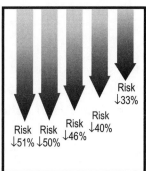

Figure 6.1 Achieving a blood pressure of under 115/75, or having your pressure that low even before starting with this plan, would make your risk much lower than it is for an average American adult.

The magnitude of the benefit is greatest if you are in your 40s or 50s, but even if you are older you benefit. That means it isn't too early to start now, and it's not too late to make sure your parents start also.

These data are from a rigorous analysis of many studies that included almost a million people who were under treatment for about a decade. Because of the huge number of people studied, the conclusions are irrefutable: people with a blood pressure under 115/75 have minimized risk.

Your goal is 115/75. You don't need to get there immediately, but you need to start right now. It's fine to take several months to get to this goal. If you have had high blood pressure for years, it may take a while to reverse. Going slowly may reduce the likelihood of any side effects of the medicines.

What if you can't get your blood pressure low enough? Even if you can lower it 20 points but don't make it to 115/75, you have markedly reduced your risk (by close to half). Getting your blood pressure lower may just take a bit more time. Blood vessels that stiffen over years take more than a few weeks to return toward normal flexibility and compliance. Wait another couple of months, then consider asking to have your dosages increased again if that is still necessary. If your pressure remains elevated after 6 to 12 months of working with your doctor, it is probably time to ask to be referred to a cardiologist or blood pressure specialist.

Cholesterol

Your doctor should order a cholesterol profile (also called a lipid profile), which includes the total cholesterol and its subtypes—high density lipoprotein (HDL cholesterol, the good stuff), low density lipoprotein (LDL cholesterol, the bad stuff) and triglycerides (modestly bad, but not as bad as high LDL or low HDL). This test is more accurate if performed after an overnight fast.

Multiple studies have demonstrated that your risk is reduced when your total cholesterol is under 160 and your LDL is under 100. Most of the early studies concentrated on total cholesterol, but this can be misleading since this value represents the sum of good (HDL) and bad (LDL and triglycerides) cholesterol. If you have a high HDL, your risk is lower, but it makes it more difficult to interpret the total cholesterol. That is why you should concentrate on your LDL.

Recent studies suggest that even if your LDL is under 100, your risks may not be minimized. There are pretty convincing data, but not yet enough for me to consider it proven, that an LDL of less than 80 reflects even lower risk for you. In fact, most cardiologists I know prefer that their LDL is less than 80. At this point, with the data available, I recommend this lower target for those who have more advanced cardiovascular disease, such as a person who already has been treated for heart disease or undergone any procedures for coronary artery disease, or has had a stroke or its warning signs.

The standard guidelines are not as strict, and that means that they are willing to leave you at higher risk of heart attacks and strokes than you should be. In Chapter 3, I describe how your risk could be 75 to 80 percent lower if you follow my guidelines instead of the standard ones, depending on your specific condition.

The lipid profile could reveal two other problems: a low level of HDL or a high triglyceride level. Both of these are important targets for treatment, but neither is treated as easily or as safely as using a statin for an elevated LDL. Using high-dose niacin can increase your HDL, but this leads to much more frequent side effects and requires closer monitoring than when using a statin. I recommend this treatment and use niacin in my practice, but it is not part of the core group of medicines for the simple reasons that niacin is not as safe or well tolerated. It requires that you work with your doctor in a way that is more complex than the core medicines in my plan require. The same problem is faced when treating high triglyceride levels, this is an important task, but one that relies on medicines that are not as safe or easily tolerated as statins (or the other core medicines of this plan).

In both cases, statins can help a little bit, so before heading off on an additional treatment or arranging appointments with other doctors, ask your doctor if your HDL and/or triglyceride levels are in the range in which the statin may be enough.

Your goal is a total cholesterol level of under 160 and an LDL of less than 100, unless you are at even higher risk; then your LDL should be under 80. By higher risk, I am referring to someone who already has coronary artery disease (diagnosed or treated now or any time in the past) or a family history of blood relatives having heart attacks when they were young. Your doctor may recommend lifestyle changes, which may sound better than taking medicine. It's worth a try, but it is unlikely to work, and even when it does, it doesn't work as well as a statin.

You should have your cholesterol profile rechecked within a couple of months, and if the effect isn't enough, have your dose increased. Although the British government thinks the risk is so low that they don't mandate checking any other blood tests, you should have your liver function tested (using a blood test) at the same time that you check your cholesterol profile, and probably according to a schedule of every three months for the first year and then every six months thereafter.

If you can't get your LDL to target, you need to ask your doctor about adding another medicine. Since your body makes most of its cholesterol while you are sleeping, taking the medicine at bedtime can help.

Diabetes Screening

Your doctor should measure your fasting blood sugar (blood glucose, to be specific) and blood HgA_{1c} levels. Most doctors routinely measure fasting blood glucose, and may even tell you that you don't need the HgA_{1c} measurement if your fasting glucose is good enough. Usually they would be right, but the tests measure your glucose metabolism in two different ways, and these are complementary ways to diagnose whether you have diabetes or the pre-diabetic condition called insulin resistance. Even though you may have a perfect blood glucose level on a particular morning, the HgA_{1c} reflects an average of your glucose control over the last three months, providing another view of your metabolism.

Your goal is an HgA_{1c} of 6 percent or less and a fasting glucose under 100. At these levels your risk is minimized since you do not have diabetes or pre-diabetes.

By the standard definitions, you have diabetes if your fasting glucose is above 125 (or an HgA_{1c} of more than 7 percent), and have pre-diabetes if your fasting glucose is above 110 (or an HgA_{1c} of more than 6 percent). The American Diabetes Association refers to pre-diabetics as having either impaired fasting glucose or impaired glucose tolerance. In either case, you're on your way to developing diabetes and need to talk to your doctor about preventative strategies. Once you have been diagnosed with diabetes (or pre-diabetes), it is recommended that you keep your HgA_{1c} under 7 percent.

By setting a goal of 7 percent, the standard guidelines are making a compromise: looser control of your diabetes in order to reduce your chances of having low blood sugar. That would be okay except for two issues. First, doctors don't seem to realize that a buffer zone has already been built in to the recommendations, which therefore tend to let you have looser diabetes control to reduce the chance of low blood sugar levels. The other problem is that the risk increases as soon as your HgA_{1c} is above 6 percent, so you are at significantly higher risk when you reach 7 percent than you need to be.

Recent studies have shown that insulin resistance can be reversed with more aggressive treatment of high blood pressure, in particular when using ACE inhibitors and the beta-blocker carvedilol. If your blood pressure isn't perfect, selecting the treatment carefully can help reverse your pre-diabetic condition.

If you are diagnosed with diabetes, you must embrace the strategy of reaching an HgA_{1c} of 6 percent or less. However, if you experience symptoms of low blood sugar as you tighten control, you may be forced to settle for less than optimal control (and perhaps settle for an HgA_{1c} of 7 percent). But before you do so, ask to see an expert who can review your approaches and hopefully find the way to reduce your sugars.

Discussing Results with Your Doctor

When your doctor reviews the results of these standard tests, he or she will be looking for results that are at the standard recommended levels, but this isn't good enough.

By telling your doctor your expectations (for optimal treatment) before the results are in, you guide the conversation towards your target, and your risk is minimized.

- "When we talked last time, I explained that I have a different attitude than I used to. I am willing to take medicines that could safely reduce my risk of a heart attack or a stroke, if the results of my tests suggest any increase in risk at all."

- "I know my risk is low, but I want it to be the lowest possible, even if it means you need to treat me even more aggressively than the standard guidelines recommend."

- "I left you some information last visit that shows how medicines such as aspirin, statins, beta-blockers and ACE inhibitors can reduce my risks, especially when they reduce my blood pressure below 115/75 and LDL cholesterol under 100."

- "I'd like to get my numbers that low, wouldn't you?"

The process should not feel intimidating. You can take the book with you and read the script or you can print out the questions on my website (http://beforeithappens.com).

If your doctor seems resistant to the whole process, you should present copies of the charts showing the extent of your risks before your doctor shows you the results. Have the charts ready that show the safety of the medicines in this plan as well, in case this question arises.

Deciding When to Treat: Risks and Side Effects

Risks are always evaluated in terms of the likelihood of something bad happening relative to the desired benefit. For example, with high-dose aspirin in people with severe high blood pressure, the risk of bleeding and suffering a disabling stroke is pretty high, and can be higher than the beneficial effect of preventing a heart attack. In that case, aspirin should not be used. However, if blood pressure is controlled and low-dose aspirin is used for someone with a 1 in 250 chance of having a heart attack within a year, the benefit becomes greater than the risk.

Similar analyses can be performed for the other medicines, but tend to be simpler than for aspirin because the other medicines are even safer. A statin is so safe that it adds no risk compared with a placebo. Any benefit (as would be the case if your LDL is above 100) becomes a net positive effect.

For ACE inhibitors, your risk could be higher if your body tends to hold on to potassium. This does not preclude treatment, but it may limit you to low doses. The risk of angioedema (explained in Chapter 4) is low. If you have vascular disease, have ever been diagnosed with coronary artery disease, diabetes or even "borderline" blood pressure, an ACE inhibitor would lower your risk of heart attacks and strokes so markedly that you would be safer taking the medicine than avoiding it.

Beta-blockers can be risky if you have severe lung disease (asthma or emphysema) or a very low heart rate. Otherwise, if you have high blood pressure, a prior heart attack or a weak heart (heart failure), the reduction in your risk of sudden death would make the decision to take a beta-blocker pretty easy.

Test	Standard Recommendation	Optimal Target
Total cholesterol	< 200	< 160
LDL cholesterol	< 100, 130 or 160	< 80 or 100
Blood pressure	< 140/90	< 115/75
Blood pressure with diabetes	< 130/80	< 115/75
Blood pressure with kidney disease	< 130/80	< 115/75
Blood pressure with heart failure	< 130/80	< 115/75
HgA$_{1c}$	< 7%	< 6%
Weight	lower	within 5% of ideal body weight

Using the Results of the Tests

Even if the results of these first three tests are within the targets of this plan, you need to get the rest of the tests performed according to the schedule in Chapter 3. However, in all likelihood, the results of these first three will not all be ideal.

If any of these are abnormal, you should have an electrocardiogram and measurement of homocysteine, CRP and BNP. If your blood pressure is above 115/75 or your BNP level is high, an echocardiogram should be performed because, in either case, thickening or weakening of your heart could have already started. For any abnormality identified, you will need to receive the medicines that are part of this plan that will enable you to achieve the targets for optimal health.

The tests must be interpreted appropriately to minimize risk. The generally accepted goals of the standard recommendations are compared with the optimal targets of this plan in the chart on page 87.

The Significance of Additional Tests

The Before It Happens Plan includes tests in addition to blood pressure, cholesterol and diabetes screening. Each of these tests can be performed in a doctor's office, and none have risk.

Homocysteine

The level of homocysteine can be lowered using B vitamins. While this would appear to make sense, studies conflict as to whether such treatment makes things better or worse. There is no doubt however, that high homocysteine levels are associated with higher risk of cardiovascular problems. Therefore, this test becomes useful for understanding your level of risk, but no specific therapy exists that is proven safe and effective (and that includes high-dose folic acid).

CRP (C-reactive protein)

CRP levels can be reduced by statins, but people with high CRP levels already meet my criteria for treatment with a statin anyway, since they either have coronary disease, diabetes or another characteristic that signifies they should be on a statin. For someone with a perfect cholesterol profile and no evidence of vascular disease who is under 50, we don't know whether taking a statin makes sense for an increased CRP. While we wait for an ongoing study to answer that question in the next few years, I would err on the side of using a statin in such a circumstance, given their overall safety.

BNP (brain naturetic peptide)

This peptide can identify people with heart failure due to a weak heart, a stiff heart or even a heart stressed by high pressure in the arteries of the lungs. An echocardiogram can distinguish between these problems.

ECG (electrocardiogram)

This is a standard test in which the minute electrical currents in your heart are recorded from sticky electrodes placed on the skin of your chest, arms and legs. Changes in the ECG (also called EKG) can be the result of structural abnormalities of the heart, or merely a normal variation without any significance. An echocardiogram can determine which.

Echocardiogram

An echocardiogram is an ultrasound test that yields moving images of the heart as it contracts and relaxes. Pressures inside the heart can be estimated and chamber sizes can be measured. If you were to be found to have a weak or dilated heart, you may require additional tests, and certainly would require treatment. The standard treatment for heart failure, as this is called, rests upon ACE inhibitors and beta-blockers. For more information about heart failure, I recommend Marc Silver's book *Living with Heart Failure.* If your heart were stiff, with thickened walls, you would need even tighter control of your blood pressure, and hopefully with optimal pressure control, the heart can return toward normal.

PART 3

Your Personalized Plan

CHAPTER 7

If You Have High Blood Pressure

IF I ASKED HOW LONG YOU HAVE HAD HIGH BLOOD PRESSURE, would you know? I'm sure you know when you started taking medicines, but you didn't think that was when it started, did you?

High blood pressure is called the silent killer for a reason. You had high blood pressure for years before you were diagnosed, and the longer you had it, the more damage it has caused to your heart, brain and kidneys. That's why high blood pressure leads to so many problems.

I hope your doctor has told you how bad high blood pressure can be, not because I want you to hear bad news, but because you can't possibly be as effective at staying healthy if you don't know what you are facing. You should know that feeling fine is no protection from high blood pressure. I don't want to make you panic, but I must establish a sense of urgency, or you may become another statistic.

In North America, the average blood pressure for people in their early 40s is above 115/75 and by the mid-50s the average reaches 125 systolic. So if your blood pressure is above average, and even 20 mm above optimum of 115/75, your risk of strokes or heart attacks is twice as high.

I hope you realize that you need to do something, starting now. You have three options to pursue: The first is the standard recommendation to change your lifestyle. If that is not sufficient or your blood pressure is really bad, the second step is to be treated according to the recent guidelines of the JNC-7(seventh cycle of the Joint National Commission), the official "bible" of blood pressure management.

The Plan for People with High Blood Pressure
....

- Your blood pressure needs to be < 115/75 (both numbers)
  - The two medicines that are first choices are ACE inhibitors and beta-blockers, because each reduces your risk more than just by lowering blood pressure (ARB may be substituted if you can't tolerate ACE inhibitors or added if blood pressure remains above 115/75 after a diuretic is added).
  - If your blood pressure remains above 115/75, a diuretic should be added.
  - If your blood pressure remains above 115/75, the calcium blocker amlodipine should be added.
  - If your blood pressure is resistant, ask your doctor to help you find a cardiologist who can help.
- Your LDL needs to be < 100, under 80 if you smoke or have a history of heart attacks in your family.
- You need to take an aspirin (81 mg) each day, starting once your blood pressure is < 140/90.

The third choice is the one supported by more convincing data than these two standards and the one that has the best of ease and effectiveness, the Before It Happens Plan.

Change Your Lifestyle: The Hard Way (But It Helps)

For the last decade, a group of investigators has pursued dietary strategies to control high blood pressure, and it works. So if you are a person who can change diets with ease, or at least someone who can stick with a diet for years, this would seem to be the way to go. Based on a program called Dietary Approaches to Stop Hypertension, the DASH diet is a program tested in scientific studies. It will not make you adopt the carnivorous lifestyle of Atkins nor the vegetarian style of Ornish, but it will lower your blood pressure; it's proven.

In fact, the DASH diet is one that makes more sense than most as a way to eat a healthy diet. And perhaps that is where it ends up doing its most good. (See Chapter 18.)

Here's the catch. Even though it works, it has a relatively modest effect. If your blood pressure starts at 145 systolic, within a couple of months of following the diet, it will be 134 systolic. That is great, but your risk is still higher than it should be. If you start at 134, it will drop near 130 systolic. The lower you start, the smaller the effect.

Does it work? Yes. Will it reduce your risk? Yes. Will it minimize your risk? No. You will need more, even if you do it right and stick with it for the long haul.

If you chose lifestyle modification, it is only *part* of the solution.

The New Guidelines for High Blood Pressure: Settling for Mediocrity

In the spring of 2003, new guidelines summarizing the state of the art for the understanding and treatment of high blood pressure were published by the seventh cycle of the Joint National Commission (JNC-7). The new guidelines were hailed by news releases from major journals and medical societies. In the media blitz surrounding these new guidelines, no one mentioned one important fact. These new guidelines set a mediocre standard.

The new guidelines aren't bad, and they are better than the last set (from 1998). But unfortunately for you, they

> ### Are you a candidate for the Before It Happens Plan?
> ••••••••••••••••••••••••••••
> Simon is 53 and understands from his doctor that his blood pressure is well controlled. Since starting on a beta-blocker, his pressure has been 135/88, below the recommended target. Simon was reassured that his chance for a heart attack, stroke or death within the next year was only 1 in 250. But his risk could be half that if we reduced his blood pressure to the optimal level according to this plan.

are ordinary and acceptable but not outstanding. After your doctor reads them, and if he or she follows them well you will be provided with a level of medical care that you could consider passable. That means they are mediocre.

Are you still willing to settle?

The guidelines do acknowledge that a blood pressure higher than 115/75 increases your risk of a heart attack, stroke, kidney failure or cardiovascular death. But that does not seem to mean to them that much needs to be done. Instead they consider you as being "pre-hypertensive" with an increased risk of developing hypertension. It is curious that they seem to forget from one page to the next about the risks that are proven to go along with even a slightly abnormal blood pressure.

The Framingham Study is one of the most famous in medicine. It took place in Framingham, Massachusetts, and when it started in 1948, the goal was to identify the risk factors for the development of cardio-vascular disease, and eventually, learn about the effectiveness of inter-vening. One of the study's insights about blood pressure was published only recently. The Framingham investigators identified those people without high blood pressure according to the standard definition, and then determined the level of risk associated with even slightly increased blood pressure. As shown in Figure 7.1, a man's risk is over 200 per-cent higher and a woman's over 500 percent higher if their blood pressure is good enough for JNC-7, compared with having blood pressure controlled to the targets of the Before It Happens Plan.

The guidelines tell your doctor to recommend lifestyle modifica-tions and use medications to lower your blood pressure under 140/90. That means that this state-of-the-art document advocates that it is okay for your risk of heart attack, stroke or cardiovascular death to be at levels twice as high as they can be with the strategies of the Before It Happens Plan.

The diagnosis of hypertension has been turned into an all-or-none concept in the minds of most doctors, when in fact the risk is gradu-

Your Are at Higher Risk of a Heart Attack, Stroke or Dying from Cardiovascular Disease with Normal or High Normal Blood Pressure Than You Could Be

Women

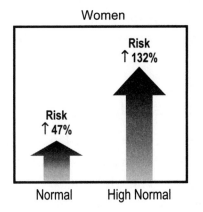

Men

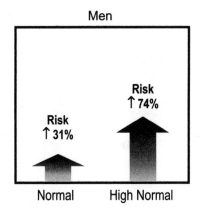

Optimal: under 130 systolic
Normal: 120-130 systolic
High Normal: 130-139 systolic

Figure 7.1 Even if your blood pressure is normal, that does not mean it is optimal. If you have normal (or high-normal) blood pressure, you are at significantly higher risk than if you had optimal pressure.

The Framingham Study has provided more insights into cardiovascular disease than any other investigation, especially as far as the importance of blood pressure. These investigators recently reported that you could be at higher risk of a heart attack or stroke even if your blood pressure seems to be okay. Although considered to be free of risk, those people with blood pressure in the normal or high-normal range were more likely to suffer a heart attack or stroke, or to die prematurely, than people with optimal blood pressure.

The figure shows the same relationships for women (box on the left) and men (right); compared to optimal blood pressure, under 115/75, even a slight increase into the 120s, though considered normal, still would be associated with increased risk of heart attacks, strokes, kidney failure and heart failure (47 percent and 31 percent bigger risk for women and men, respectively, than if the blood pressure were less than 120 systolic.

ally increasing as soon as your pressure goes above the ideal of 115/75. The early stages are the time to intervene most effectively, as your pressure is going higher, not after it reaches some extreme value.

Doctors consider a patient whose blood pressure is 134/88 as fine, while another person with a blood pressure of 138/92 is borderline and a third with a pressure of 142/94 is hypertensive. There is little difference between these three measurements, each indicating increased risk.

The Easy Way (Safe and Scientific as Well)

The Before It Happens Plan shares some of the views of JNC-7, the newest guidelines about high blood pressure. Both plans acknowledge that lifestyle modification is not likely to be enough for most people and that more than one medicine will generally be needed to lower your blood pressure to target.

Both plans agree that optimal blood pressure is 115/75 or less; they disagree about what to do for you. However, the JNC-7 guidelines are willing to accept treatment that gets you only part of the way there, considering it adequate to leave you at twice the risk of a heart attack or stroke. In contrast, the Before It Happens Plan gets your blood pressure under 115/75, minimizing your risk.

The standard approach is to get your blood pressure to 135/85. Your risk is twice as high at that level as it would be at the target of

---

What is the blood pressure at which your risk is minimized?

The results are the same in every study; standard targets are too high.

Seven Communities Study (1970s):	<120/77
Framingham Study (2001):	<120/80
Prospective Studies Collaboration (2003):	<115/75
The JNC-7 conclusion:	<115/75

this program, 115/75 (see Figure 6.1 in Chapter 6). Is leaving your risk twice as high as it could be good enough for you?

The Benefits of the Plan

Let's think about this for a moment. Having high blood pressure increases your risk of a stroke, heart attack, kidney failure and death. Treatments exist (and are the ones in this program) that are proven safe and are proven to lower your blood pressure (safety records are reviewed in Chapter 4). Studies prove that this plan will lower your risk. What are you waiting for?

There are times doctors will argue over which medicine is best, and it is true your care should be individualized. However, there are several medicines that are proven in study after study to be superior (and others that sometimes work and sometimes may not be as good). ACE inhibitors and beta-blockers provide additional benefits, beyond merely lowering blood pressure.

It's okay if your doctor prefers to start with a diuretic; that is supported by scientific data. However, a diuretic is not enough even if it lowers your blood pressure under 115/75. Diuretics do reduce your risk of heart attacks and strokes, but they do so by lowering blood pressure, and do not provide additional benefits in terms of the plaques in your arteries.

Compared to another type of blood pressure medicine, calcium channel blockers, ACE inhibitors reduce your risk of heart attacks even when they are used at doses that don't lower blood pressure as much. Beta-blockers reduce the risk of sudden death. These are effects that are so important that these medicines deserve to be the first agents used.

Implementing the Plan

Once you are diagnosed with hypertension, make sure your doctor considers the possibility of a reversible cause. Although very few people with high blood pressure have a reversible cause that can be identified and treated, it is worth asking.

- "How can we make sure that I don't have a reversible and potentially curable cause for my high blood pressure?"

Also tell your doctor that you plan to improve your lifestyle but realize that even your best-intended commitment won't be enough over the years to come. Exercise, weight loss and salt (sodium) restriction will help but are difficult to keep up for years. It is unlikely that you will be able to change habits that you have had for the last 40 or 50 years and not revert back to them. Besides, the amount of impact from lifestyle change is relatively small, so you will need medicines anyway to reach your goals.

If your doctor is constantly telling you to change your lifestyle and you cannot do it, then you are going to dread each medical appointment and are unlikely to feel good about the relationship you have with that doctor. That means that it will be increasingly difficult for the two of you to work as partners towards your healthcare. That is why you need to set limits starting now.

- "I will work to change my lifestyle as a way to lower my blood pressure, but I will probably be like most people, either unable to stick to it or able to improve my blood pressure only a little bit, probably only a few millimeters."

An example of how to ask about blood pressure management is included in Chapter 6, in the section describing how to discuss results with your doctor. You could use these questions, omitting the parts about cholesterol levels and statins, unless that also is relevant to you. Alternatively, consider these.

- "I am reading a book that explains that the most recent guidelines for blood pressure management, referred to as JNC-7, report an even lower level for an ideal blood pressure. The document points out that the best research indicates that a blood pressure of less than 115/75 puts me at the lowest possible risk, about half the risk of having a heart attack or stroke compared to a typical blood pressure goal of 135/85."

- "The book also points out that ACE inhibitors and beta-blockers are incredibly safe medicines to use to reach these blood pressure levels, sometimes with the addition of a diuretic."
- "Since my risk would be minimized with such a treatment plan, is there any reason why I should not be given these safe medicines to avoid the disability associated with a heart attack or stroke?"

The Medicines That Work

While I personally advocate lifestyle changes, which you will read about in Chapters 16, 17 and 18, this is not the primary focus of this plan because lifestyle changes don't work well enough; they are too hard for most, and not potent enough for the remainder.

As someone with high blood pressure or borderline blood pressure, you need to help your doctor to get your blood pressure to 115/75. The medications that can do that most effectively with the greatest benefit to reducing the risk of heart attack, strokes or premature death are the ACE inhibitors and beta-blockers. In general, one would be started before the other with gradually increasing dosage towards the maximum tolerated. Depending on your blood pressure, the increases in the doses could occur over several days or even a few months. Each of these two medicines, ACE inhibitors and beta-blockers, are effective in reducing blood pressure but also provide added benefits.

The ACE inhibitors can stabilize plaques of fat in your arteries that are prone to rupture, and, by doing so, these agents can reduce the risks of heart attacks and sudden death. In addition, ACE inhibitors can reduce your risk of developing diabetes, can protect your kidneys if you have diabetes, and can slightly improve glucose control in diabetics by increasing the sensitivity to insulin. For these reasons, ACE inhibitors provide more than mere blood pressure lowering effects, and that is why they are the key components of this plan.

In addition to their blood pressure–lowering effect, beta-blockers can reduce the risk of heart attacks, can improve the function of the blood vessels, and can reduce sudden death both in patients with hypertension as well as those who have had a heart attack. Because of these added benefits, beta-blockers are also a prominent part of the plan. If your blood pressure has not reached 115/75 after a few months of treatment, the structural changes in your arteries are unlikely to reverse completely, so additional therapies should be instituted.

Although not a key part of the plan, thiazide diuretics also reduce blood pressure. Although diuretics are thought of as medicines that will make you urinate, when thiazide diuretics are used at their approved doses, the effect tends to be very mild and the increase in urination is only noticeable for the first few days of use. Clinical trials have proven that long-term use of diuretics does reduce blood pressure.

As a final step for a person who cannot get to a blood pressure of 115/75, the calcium channel blocker amlodipine should be considered. Calcium channel blockers are not interchangeable. Amlodipine is an effective drug for reducing blood pressure, and it has the largest safety record of any calcium blocker. It is the only one showing consistency of effect with large numbers of patients studied. In contrast, for other calcium blockers, some studies are favorable while others are unfavorable. The consistency in safety is the reason amlodipine stands apart from the other calcium blockers.

Once your blood pressure is controlled either to a level of 115/75, at least a 20 point drop from where it started, or to a level consistently below 140/90, therapy with low-dose aspirin should be initiated. While many have advocated doses between 75 mg and 325 mg, the lower doses appear to have the same beneficial effects while they also have a lower risk of bleeding. Therefore, my standard dose would be 81 mg once daily.

As a person with high blood pressure, even borderline blood pressure, you certainly have vascular disease. Therefore, if you are also a smoker, have diabetes or a have family history of coronary artery disease, a statin should be instituted to lower your cholesterol. The target would be to maintain an LDL-cholesterol of under 100. In fact, if your LDL is above 100 and you have no other risk factor other than your hypertension, you should start a statin as well. The two agents with the largest track record and greatest potency are simvastatin and atorvastatin, although pravastatin and lovastatin also are very effective. Because pravastatin is not as potent, I tend to use this drug primarily in people who have a history of liver disease or who take medicines for other conditions that are heavily metabolized in the liver.

If you are over 50, controlling blood pressure, even to optimal levels, is not enough. Read the Chapters 14 and 15 for men and women without a specific diagnosis to understand how to lower your risk further, as a complementary strategy to achieving optimal blood pressure.

Is "White Coat" Hypertension the Same As Real Hypertension?

White coat hypertension describes what happens to many people when visiting the doctor. Worried about what will happen, you get a little nervous, and because your cardiovascular system is more sensitive to the stress, your blood pressure rises, as much as 30 points in some studies.

Is "white coat" hypertension the same as real hypertension? The guidelines say "no" but the scientific evidence says "almost." People with white coat hypertension don't have the same risk of strokes or heart attacks as those with blood pressure that is always high, but they are almost as bad off. If you have white coat hypertension, the structure of your heart is changing, developing hypertrophy (muscle thickening) that can be detected on an echocardiogram, a sign that your risk of a heart attack or stroke is getting higher.

Most doctors were taught that white coat hypertension does not need to be treated because the pressure was only increased transiently in the doctor's office, an environment different from normal every day life. But is it?

Hopefully, you live somewhere and have a lifestyle different from most other people. Perhaps you do not face traffic congestion on your way to and from work. Perhaps you stay completely relaxed as you look through your monthly bills and never get frustrated or feel stress when your children need your help with their homework after dinner (while you need to recover from a busy day). You may have plenty of time and energy to make sure your marriage and family relationships are perfect and stress free.

On the other hand, maybe you have stressful times throughout the day, not necessarily big ones, but enough to raise your blood pressure as if there were a doctor in a white coat standing next to you.

Since your blood vessels and heart are transiently exposed to high blood pressure, studies to evaluate the impact long term are crucial, yet not included in the discussion of the blood pressure guidelines. Studies have shown that people with white coat hypertension develop changes in their heart that are even more severe than people with mildly high blood pressure. These changes include left ventricular hypertrophy of your heart, a sign that your risk is even higher.

If you have white coat hypertension, you are welcome to adjust your lifestyle, but if that doesn't work, you need the medicines in the Before It Happens Plan. (If you do figure out how to change your life enough, email me so I can tell my patients and professional colleagues, and use the information for myself.)

The Reality of High Blood Pressure

- Get your blood pressure taken in both arms at least once to make sure there isn't a major discrepancy.
- Keep track of your own blood pressure. Write it down after each medical appointment. Because most of us see several types of doctors, all of whom check blood pressure, we're in the best position to make sure our blood pressure isn't on the increase.

Structural Changes of the Heart
Occur If Your Blood Pressure Is Always High
and Even If It Is Only High Sometimes

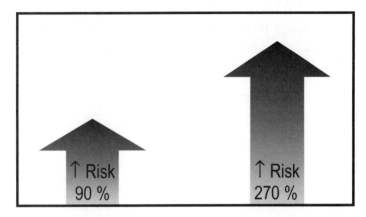

Figure 7.2 Some people have good blood pressure whenever it is measured, while others have blood pressure that is good almost all the time. People with "White Coat Hypertension" can have their pressure jump up by 30 points or more whenever the doctor comes into the room in his or her long white coat.

Most of these people aren't treated with medicines, but they should be. You know that having high pressure all the time, whether mild or severe, will lead to structural changes in the heart that can be difficult to reverse. Most doctors don't realize that even people with white coat hypertension eventually will develop structural heart disease, with a 90 percent higher likelihood of having such changes detectable by a standard echocardiogram. These kinds of changes, when present, mean that your risk of a heart attack or stroke has increased, with the risk of stroke dramatically higher.

- "White coat" hypertension isn't just a temporary thing; the condition indicates a tendency toward high blood pressure. Take it seriously.

• Tell your doctor you are willing to take medication in order to get your blood pressure down to 115/75.

• Your doctor will make the final selection of medicines, and she or he may consider an ACE inhibitor, a beta-blocker, and/or a diuretic.

• Adjust your lifestyle as you can. Smokers should stop smoking, and you need to watch your cholesterol to guard against other heart problems.

CHAPTER 8

If You Have High Cholesterol

UNLESS YOUR CHOLESTEROL IS PERFECT, YOU HAVE SOME work to do. Each year, your risk of a heart attack or stroke increases, and it rises faster as your cholesterol level increases. The fat-filled plaques are becoming more widespread in your arteries and more vulnerable to rupture. Even a small increase in cholesterol can markedly increase your risk. For example, the standard recommendations say that for most of you, an LDL of 125 is good control. But several studies show that this would not minimize your risk. Figure 4.2 in Chapter 4 is one of several illustrations that show that your risk isn't minimized until your LDL is well under 100.

You know you must do something, and start now. You have two options, the hard way and the easy way. It's your choice.

Change Your Lifestyle: The Hard Way

Ready to be a vegetarian? When will you be scheduling your hour each day for stress management, including meditation, stretches, relaxation techniques and directed or receptive imagery? Will you exercise for 30 minutes each day or one hour three times a week? How can you make sure you are eating the right mixture of foods, ones without saturated fat but with the right balance of proteins?

I am overwhelmed just listing the questions. These are the major components used in Dean Ornish's program, which is the best studied and most effective lifestyle intervention program for treating heart disease. Its main problem is exemplified by the observation that I have met only one person who could change to this diet successfully.

The Ornish Program Dietary Goals

	Typical Diet	Ornish Diet
Fat	40–50%	10%
Carbohydrates	25–35%	70–75%
Protein	25%	15–25%
Cholesterol	400–500 mg	5 mg

About a hundred people enrolled in the scientific studies of his program and each continued their heart medicines while in the study. At the time of the studies, in the late 1980s, a strong case existed for optimal cholesterol and blood pressure control, but the tools were not as well defined as they are now. Yes, statins, beta-blockers and ACE inhibitors were available, but at that time no one realized how safe these medicines were, and certainly there was not nearly the evidence to support their effectiveness.

For several weeks, while living in a spa-like environment, they received meals prepared by accomplished chefs (this was not institutional food). Immersing themselves in this controlled lifestyle (one radically different than yours or mine) changed these people. Somehow they managed to stick with the diet and lifestyle even after returning to the real world. The participants had their cholesterol levels drop by 20 percent and their LDL (the bad one) by 30 percent. Despite a slight drop in HDL (the good one, which you would want to increase), their symptoms of angina improved and the blockages in their coronary arteries improved. Such data are cause for optimism about the likelihood that heart attacks can be prevented, but no study has shown that to be the case.

The Ornish program works: but can you really make it work for you? If so, you should do it. But even if you do, realize that the participants were not cured. Their cholesterol levels were not optimal and they still had plaques in their arteries despite all their hard work, and they remained at risk.

Most people can't completely give up the idea of going out to a nice restaurant, occasionally ordering a filet mignon or perhaps dessert. The Ornish program isn't easy to follow. Fortunately, there is a more practical approach, one that you *can* follow and which is proven to reduce risk.

The Before It Happens Plan: The Easy Way

The Before It Happens Plan is the easy and safe way to stay alive and healthy, and it's the most effective approach too. Statins safely lower your cholesterol level, and more importantly, prevent new plaques from forming in your arteries and stabilize the plaques you already have (making them less vulnerable to rupture).

The Plan for People with High Cholesterol
• •

- Take a statin to get your LDL-cholesterol < 100, or < 80 if you need aggressive treatment* (this will lower your total cholesterol to 160 unless you are lucky enough to have high levels of good cholesterol (HDL).

- Talk to your doctor about treatment if your HDL-cholesterol is < 40 (men) or < 50 (women).

- If you have a sibling, parent or child who has had a heart attack, angioplasty or bypass surgery, you should start with the Before It Happens Plan at least 10 years younger than the age at which they were first diagnosed, and get your LDL < 80.

- Talk to your doctor about treatment if your triglyceride level is > 150.

- Talk to your doctor about taking an aspirin (81 mg) and an ACE inhibitor if you need aggressive treatment.*

*Aggressive treatment is needed if you have had a heart attack, an angioplasty, a bypass; you get chest pains; you are a diabetic; you are over 50 and smoke; or you are over 50 and have a first-degree relative with heart disease.

Get your cholesterol profile checked (do it after an overnight fast and make sure that LDL, HDL, triglycerides, C-reactive protein and homocysteine are measured as discussed in Chapter 3). If your results are not optimal, tell your doctor you want to be treated with a statin. Then take your statin every night before bed. You will get a blood test every three months for the first year, and if they look good, your doctor will probably change it to every six months.

You're done. You would then have lowered your risk of a heart attack, stroke or premature death by more than 25 percent, well on your way to the overall 50 percent reduction in risk once all the components of the plan are in place. Each step is simple, safe and effective, based on volumes of scientific studies.

Your statin isn't steak insurance, permitting you to live on a high-cholesterol diet; it is life assurance, permitting you to live longer and be healthier.

You should not stop trying to improve your lifestyle, but it is pretty neat that this pill each day can keep you alive.

Would You Benefit?

Yes.

If your cholesterol is not optimal, you are at higher risk than you need to be. Your targets are total cholesterol under 160, LDL choles-

---

Are you a candidate for the Before It Happens Plan?
••

Robert is 46, and had an LDL cholesterol of 165. His father had open-heart surgery in his late 70s, but Robert thought that didn't matter, after all, his father was not a young man. However, Robert's wife forced him to come to my office, and helped me convince Robert to start on a statin (after he spent three months unsuccessfully trying to change his diet). Robert's risk was 1 in 200 of a heart attack, stroke or death in the next year, but the Before It Happens Plan reduced his risk by more than 80 percent.

Lower LDL Level Reduces Your Likelihood
of Suffering Heart Attack
(or the Warning Signs of a Heart Attack)

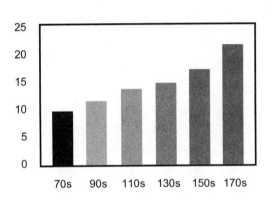

Percent
of People with
a Heart Attack
or Warning Signs

LDL Level

Figure 8.1   The lower your LDL level, the lower your risk of heart attack. Several studies have shown that getting your LDL below 80 is the most beneficial for people at the highest risk.

In this study, called 4S, people with an LDL in the 70s (black bar) benefited the most, without any evidence of a higher risk of side effects.

terol under 100 and HDL above 40 (for men) or 50 (for women). If you have had a heart attack, any procedures or operations to fix blockages, smoke, have diabetes or narrowings in the arteries anywhere in your body (including your legs), then your LDL should be under 80. If you are lucky enough to have a very high HDL level, your total cholesterol could be above 160, so use the LDL level as the ultimate target.

Your doctor probably thinks that you have to have a very high LDL to warrant treatment with a statin. That is only part of the truth. The worse your cholesterol is, the easier it is to prove that there is benefit. But now we have enough data to know that your risk is higher than it

> ## You can calculate your risk of a heart attack right now
> Go to http://hin.nhlbi.nih.gov/atpiii/calculator.asp?usertype=prof and answer the questions using the results from your most recent blood test and doctor appointment. The result will be your risk over the next 10 years. In the text, I generally refer to your risk within a year, which is derived from this website set up by the National Institutes of Health.

needs to be, even if your cholesterol level seems to be good enough. Taking a statin can help you avoid that heart attack and stay alive.

Worried about the risk of taking a medicine? That is good; you should be worried enough to ask about the safety record. Each of the medicines in this plan, and particularly statins, are incredibly safe. Scientific studies have proven that there is more cause for concern about taking anti-oxidant vitamins than there is about taking a statin. You can read about the safety record in Chapter 4.

You are safer taking a statin than trying to live without one.

If you have diabetes or vascular disease, you must be on a statin as long as your cholesterol level is greater than 135, in order to stay alive. If you are a smoker, you should follow this same approach, since your arteries are probably just as bad and your risk just as high.

Start Now: You Already Have Heart Disease

In Chapter 2 I described the process of plaque development and increasing risk of catastrophic plaque rupture. The process starts in our 20s, and eventually the amount of fat in the walls of the arteries is enough that the immune system is activated to clean up the mess.

This protective mechanism backfires in the long run. When the cells of the immune system pass through the caps of the plaques and attempt to digest the fat, they leave behind small cracks in the caps that cover the plaques, cracks that compromise the strength of the caps. As more cells invade, the size of the plaques increases, pushing up against the delicate caps, like pimples ready to burst. If the caps stretch to the point of rupture, the fat and active immune cells are exposed to the blood, and a clot forms almost immediately.

The formation of a blood clot is the body's protective method of sealing off this fatty material, but this backfires as well, since the clot itself can totally clog the vessel and cause a heart attack or sudden heart arrhythmia, either of which could prove fatal.

When you start to form plaques in your arteries, two main types can develop: In one, the plaques block a lot but not all of the blood flow (even without a rupture). The others don't affect blood flow at all because they only fill up 20 to 30 percent of the artery. These are the ones that are vulnerable to rupture.

The big plaques cause symptoms (chest pains and shortness of breath) and are easy to detect on standard testing. The smaller plaques cannot be detected, but are the ones that pose the danger. If you have a plaque rupture, you would feel pain or pressure of a heart attack, or perhaps shortness of breath or nausea (see Appendix A), and you could have only seconds, minutes or hours to live. Over 250,000 people die suddenly without warning due to an acute blockage in one of the arteries of the heart.

These risks are real. Ask around. Most people in their 50s can think of at least one friend or one famous person who has died suddenly. Statistically, sudden death occurs in more people each year than are diagnosed with breast cancer and colon cancer combined.

There is no controversy about when the fatty plaques start. Over 75 percent of war casualties and young trauma victims have coronary artery plaques, and a fifth have plaques that are extensive. Plaques can also be seen when people undergo a special type of cardiac catheterization, with insertion of an ultrasound wire into the arteries of the heart (this is a bit riskier than a regular catheterization). As shown in Figure 2.2 in Chapter 2, 60 percent of people in their 30s, 70 percent in their 40s and over 85 percent in their 50s have significant fatty plaques in a major coronary artery.

The scientific evidence leaves no doubt; we are all going to develop fat deposits and blockages in the arteries of our heart, or coronary artery disease.

You can't start too early. The ideal time is before middle age, depending on your medical condition, generally in your 40s, when most have heart disease (even though few of us can tell) and when the disease is still largely reversible. Statistically speaking, starting treatment in middle age has the greatest impact on society, as opposed to the approach currently advocated by our health system of waiting for more advanced disease, which is more common with people in their 60s and 70s. It's good to start older people on treatment, too, just later than ideal.

Already you and I are way behind, and need to work hard to catch up with the disease. This plan provides an easy and powerful way to close the gap and reduce your risk.

Benefits of Therapy

Maybe you already knew that your cholesterol was a big problem. Most people know they need to "eventually do something" but don't feel great urgency. There are two reasons you need to feel that sense of urgency. First, your risk is high. And second, there is something safe and easy to do that will dramatically lower your risk. A statin will

Even the NCEP/ATP-3 report understands that starting treatment early is a more powerful approach to controlling heart disease:

" . . . a 10% reduction in serum cholesterol level attained at age 40 yields a reduction in relative risk for coronary heart disease of 50% at age 40, whereas a 10% cholesterol reduction gives only a 20% reduction in risk if begun at age 70. This finding implies that the greatest long-term benefit is attained by early intervention; conversely, later intervention yields lesser benefit in risk reduction." (p II-7) keep you alive and prevent disabling events. (There is even some data that suggest it could lower your risk of Alzheimer's.)

In Chapter 4, I reviewed several major trials using statins. There are hundreds of studies demonstrating benefits. These studies show that the benefits far exceed the risk of rare problems, including allergic reactions, and liver or muscle irritations. Statins reduce the risk of a stroke or disabling heart attack, and extend your life. They have practically no side effects. No doubt about it, you are safer taking one than avoiding them.

Take Control and Make It Happen

You already understand the strategy of the Before It Happens Plan. You will explain to your doctor how you want to be treated in a way that makes it easy for your doctor to change his or her approach for your benefit.

First, you must make sure that your doctor is thinking about what to do based on the optimal benefits for you and not for society. To do this, your doctor needs to think about your risks with treatment as compared to your risks without treatment. This comparison requires awareness of scientific data that are not familiar to all doctors. You will provide this data to make the decision making process one that focuses on you.

To start, remind your doctor that your goal is to have minimal risk.

- "I know that the cholesterol treatment guidelines set specific goals for my cholesterol level, but you and I both know that these guidelines are largely based on the cost-benefit to society of treatment. Since our goal right now is the optimal benefit-to-risk ratio *for me,* and not society, I wanted to talk to you about getting my cholesterol profile to *optimal* levels."

- "I visited an NIH website where I calculated my risk of a heart attack or cardiac death over the next few years, and it was a lot higher than I expected. I know I am low risk, but I want to be at the *lowest risk.*"

- "This is a reasonable goal, at least in theory, don't you agree?"

You would pause to allow your doctor to nod or say yes, or even just to let him or her think about what you just said. The statements leading up to this question would be considered quite reasonable by any rational person.

- "I am reading this book that says that many scientific studies have shown that statins are incredibly safe and reduce the risk of plaques rupturing, which is the primary trigger for a heart attack."
- "I am not sure if a study has ever been performed on people exactly like me, but is there any reason why I wouldn't want to take any medicine that is so safe and can keep me alive? A statin makes a lot of sense to me."

You have now established that you understand the issues of risk-benefit and cost-benefit ratios, the importance of drug safety and the power of the statin to save your life. But you have also done one other important thing. You have become an informed, articulate advocate, and now your doctor has to decide whether to talk you out of this, or to move in the obvious direction of considering whether you have a reason for not taking a statin. Believe me, if your LDL cholesterol is high; even above 100, your doctor should realize you should be on a statin.

Who Should Not Take a Statin?

Statins are not recommended for people who have active and significant liver disease. Statins are also not usually given to patients who have an elevated total cholesterol due to very high levels of good cholesterol (this is unusual). If that is the case and your total cholesterol is above 160 or 200, but your LDL is below 100, things are good enough and you probably should not be on a statin.

What if your doctor hesitates?

Your doctor may need some time to figure out how he or she is going to handle change, looking for a way that doesn't make him or her look bad for not considering this in the past. You can give your doctor the chance to reevaluate at the next appointment, but the next appointment should be within 3 to 6 months.

Figure 8.2 shows the effects of statins demonstrated in the major clinical trials that led to their widespread use. There are other studies with other statins, and the effects are consistent for the four statins used in these studies (pravastatin, simvastatin, atorvastatin and lovastatin).

When you show this table to your doctor, draw attention to the last two columns, highlighting the HPS study patients who started with an LDL under 116 and those who started below 100. In both cases, the patients benefited by the same relative risk reduction as those who started with a higher LDL level.

This is a drug that reduces your risk dramatically. (See Figure 8.3.)

- "The reason I am so interested in starting on a statin, even though in general I do not like to take extra medicines, is summarized in this table." (See Table 4.2 in Chapter 4. It is a good idea to point to it to make sure he or she sees it.)

- "The Heart Protection Study included a lot of diabetics, but also a lot of people with vascular disease. When the data from the Heart Protection Study were reviewed for those patients with low (<116) or very low (< 100) LDL levels, their risk was reduced markedly as well. I would like to take such a safe medicine if it can lower my risk too."

If you have an elevated cholesterol level, and your doctor has not handed you a prescription by now, or has not explained why you are the exception, you have another problem. Your doctor does not seem willing or able to treat you for optimal health. Don't make a scene, but

Statins Reduce Your Risk
of Heart Attacks, Strokes and Premature Death
Whether You Start with a Very High LDL or a Very Low LDL

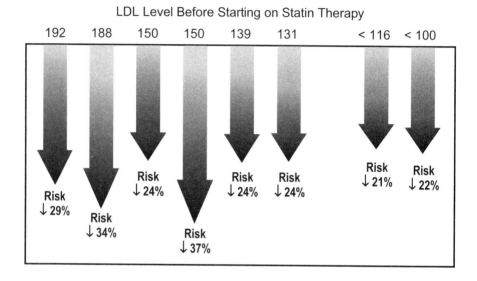

Figure 8.2 The relative benefit of a statin is consistent; no matter how high or low your LDL starts out; taking a standard dose will reduce your risk by 20 to 30 percent.

At the right side of the figure is the effect of a statin in groups of people whose LDL is reasonably low prior to starting treatment, less than 116 or less than 100. Statin therapy reduced risk significantly in both of these groups, too.

get yourself to another doctor to find out if the problem was a simple communication block, or whether you need a new doctor.

Perhaps you have a low HDL or high triglycerides, with or without elevated LDL. I focus on LDL because of its relationship to risk and because we have potent and safe ways to fix the problem. However, statins do relatively little for HDL or triglyceride levels, so an additional drug may be warranted. The medications for these problems, when taken with a statin, increase your risk of liver and muscle irrita-

Aggressively Lowering Your LDL
Can Reduce Your Risk Markedly
(risks calculated for people 45–64 years old)

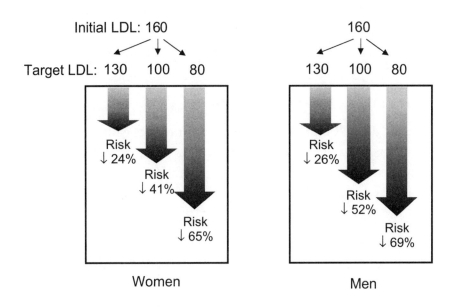

Figure 8.3 Based on the Framingham and Atherosclerosis Risk in the Community Studies, the effect of lowering cholesterol can be estimated based upon the amount that the LDL level is reduced.

A woman or man at moderate risk, a middle aged-smoker, for example, would have cut risk by 24 to 26 percent by following the standard guidelines. In contrast, the Before It Happens Plan would cut risk by 41 to 52 percent.

If you are low risk with an LDL of 160, this plan will cut your risk by 41 to 52 percent.

If you are at high risk, and need aggressive treatment, your risk would be cut by 65 to 69 percent.

These effects are realized by selecting treatment goals that safely minimize your risk.

tion. If combination therapy makes sense, see your doctor or a consultant who is experienced at treating this combination in a low-risk fashion.

You could give the book away at this point, to let someone else benefit from it, but first you should review the chapters that describe other risks you may face, each with a treatment strategy that will dovetail nicely with your statin, each of which will extend your life.

The Reality of High Cholesterol

- Even a small increase in cholesterol increases your risk of heart attack or stroke, so now is the time to bring down your cholesterol numbers.

- A problem with cholesterol leaves you vulnerable to plaque rupture, which sometimes results in sudden death.

- Your total cholesterol target should be under 160, and LDL cholesterol under 100 and HDL above 40 for men and above 50 for women.

- Your doctor can prescribe a statin, with a target LDL of under 80 if you are at the highest risk, to prevent a disabling event.

- For optimum health, adjust your eating habits to lower your cholesterol intake.

CHAPTER 9

If You Already Have Heart Disease

I WAS RETURNING FROM A MEETING A FEW MONTHS AGO, and I struck up a conversation with my cab driver. Frank was in his mid-60s and a bit overweight. He asked me what I did, and when I told him I was a cardiologist, he started telling me his medical history. He had had an angioplasty recently and was quite pleased that his chest pains were gone. He was unsure of his blood pressure or cholesterol levels but was taking an aspirin a day.

When I asked whether his doctor had discussed any other medicines or treatments for his coronary artery disease, he was perplexed: "Why should he? I don't have the problem any more." In fact, he had two problems: coronary artery disease and ignorance. He was effectively robbing himself of life-saving treatments.

By the time you know you have heart disease, your risk of a heart attack, stroke, or premature death is substantial. In Frank's case, his pains were caused by a severe narrowing of one of the arteries in his heart, but he almost certainly had more problems spread throughout his coronary arteries, since heart disease doesn't occur only in one spot. Anyone who has had an angioplasty, a heart attack or a bypass operation has many plaques throughout the arteries, but most won't be enough of a blockage for your doctor to detect on any of the standard tests. They will be the small, fat-filled, vulnerable ones. Because these plaques are so unpredictable, Frank was a walking time bomb.

Could you have many vulnerable plaques?

You should answer "yes" if you:

- Had an angioplasty, heart attack or bypass operation
- Have a history of heart disease in your family
- Have diabetes
- Are a smoker
- Are over 50 (or post-menopausal) and have high cholesterol (LDL > 100 or total cholesterol > 160), high blood pressure (> 115/75) or are overweight (> 10% above ideal)

If you could have vulnerable plaques, you need to be treated very aggressively. I hope you have already adopted a healthier lifestyle, because you know that exercising and watching your eating habits help. Unfortunately, a healthy lifestyle doesn't protect you as much as you may think. The Before It Happens Plan will reduce your risk by 50 percent or more whether or not you can change your lifestyle.

The Plan for People with Heart Disease

- Your LDL needs to be < 80.
- Your blood pressure needs to be < 115/75 (both numbers)
- You need an ACE inhibitor to protect your blood vessels.
- You need a beta-blocker to prevent sudden death.
- You need to take an aspirin (81 mg) each day.
- You need your HDL > 40 (man) or > 50 (woman).
- If you have had an angioplasty or stent, you need to take clopidogrel.
- If you have diabetes, you need your HgA_{1c} to be < 6%.

What Is Happening to Your Body

For most people, cardiovascular disease starts in the blood vessels and eventually leads to damage to your heart, brain and other vital organs.

Threading through bad Manhattan traffic on the way to my hospital from the airport in Frank's cab, Frank and I had quite a bit of time to chat, and the experience gave rise to an analogy that I thought might help Frank—and you.

Anyone who has been to New York City knows that almost every road has more volume than it can handle, and the challenge of driving through the city is exacerbated because of the number of potholes that dot the roadways. (Repairs seem to get underway five or ten years after the problems are already unbearable.) As we found ourselves crawling through Manhattan traffic, seemingly hitting a pothole every 10 feet, it occurred to me that this was analogous to how blood was flowing through Frank's heart. The heavy traffic being slowed by potholes was similar to Frank's blood trying to make its way through plaque-lined arteries. Of course, the blood would eventually get to the heart muscle, just as I would eventually get to my office, albeit slowly. But if Frank exerted himself, making his heart need more oxygen and

---

Are you a candidate for the Before It Happens Plan?

Jim is 55 and an avid runner. Three years ago, he had a heart attack and required an angioplasty with a stent. He's back to running, feeling confident on his aspirin and statin. Jim's risk of dying before he reaches 65 is over 50 percent. Adding an ACE inhibitor and a beta-blocker could lower his risk by 60 percent, even though he thinks he doesn't even have coronary artery disease anymore.

nutrients, the blood would have a tough time making the delivery fast enough.

Plaques—and potholes—also make us vulnerable: At any moment, a plaque could rupture and stop blood flow, just as a small pothole can open up and form a deep and wide gash in the road, big enough to damage a car's front axle. Frank was at risk of sudden death just as his car was at risk of sudden breakdown.

Bumping along in the back of the cab, I realized that if Frank could recognize that he was not cured, then he could take the first steps toward getting better by talking to his doctor about the Before It Happens Plan. If Frank wouldn't admit he still had a problem, he wouldn't be able to move forward successfully—even with the simple steps of this plan.

If, like Frank, you have had an angioplasty or stent, you should notice significant improvement in your symptoms. However, despite the fact that large studies prove these procedures improve symptoms, they are not proven to reduce your risk of dying except when they are performed in the middle of a heart attack.

Fixing one pothole on the road doesn't make for smooth driving in Manhattan, and putting one stent in Frank's vessel doesn't restore normal function or eliminate his risk. If you have heart disease, you, too, need to ask for aggressive treatment. By implementing this plan, the cardiovascular disease affecting you can be reversed, and your risk of a heart attack, stroke or premature death is markedly reduced.

What about Additional Testing?

Sometimes a doctor will order additional testing to verify whether or not a person has heart disease. I hope I've convinced you by now that if you have "borderline" blood pressure or cholesterol or "little" chest pains, you have heart disease. To consider going on this plan, no additional testing is necessary.

Even if your doctor orders a stress test and then tries to reassure you that you have no severe blockages, you now should realize that most heart attacks are caused by the rupturing of small plaques—the types that are not detected by a stress test. Tell your doctor that you understand this, and that you expect to receive optimal therapy to prevent additional events, even if it requires medical therapy. Most doctors I know don't take the time to explain this because most patients are resistant to taking more medicines. However, if you've read this far, then you obviously understand that if a medicine can save your life, you should know about it. Tell your doctor you are interested in any treatment that can keep you alive. When you do so, the data will point directly to the components of the Before It Happens Plan.

Recent studies have proven the usefulness of additional blood tests to determine whether you are at even higher risk of a heart attack—specifically, measuring your blood levels of homocysteine and C-reactive protein (CRP). If your levels of either are elevated, you are at higher risk. But no study has demonstrated that doing anything about the blood levels does you any good.

Homocysteine is easy to lower by using a combination of B vitamins, and one study showed that such a strategy can keep your arteries open after having a stent placed. However, a more recent study, performed just as carefully, showed that the B vitamin treatment made the stents more likely to fail. Because there is conflict in the data, no one can be sure that taking B vitamins to lower homocysteine levels is a smart idea. Therefore I do not recommend B vitamins routinely.

CRP levels are widely measured, but there is no study suggesting that lowering your level is possible or beneficial. Statins are the only treatment that can lower CRP levels, but you probably needed to be on one anyway.

In the coming years, we will know more about possible ways to treat someone who has high homocysteine or CRP. For now, you should stick to those medicines definitively proven.

If you've had a heart attack, discussing the following issues with your doctor can save your life.

- "The American Heart Association says that my risk of dying within 8 years of my heart attack is 50 percent."

- "I am reading this book that says that my risk of another heart attack or stroke is minimized if my blood pressure is under 115/75 and my LDL is less than 80."

- "It also says that the HOPE and EUROPA trials and the Heart Protection Study proved that ACE inhibitors and statins cut my risk even if I don't have high blood pressure or cholesterol."

- "The book also says that the risk of sudden death for people like me who have had a heart attack, especially if my heart is weak, is reduced significantly by beta-blockers."

- "How can I make sure I am taking these medicines that seem so well suited to keep me alive for years to come?"

If you've undergone an angioplasty, like Frank, or a bypass operation, add the following issues to the discussion:

- "I am reading a book that says that even though the blockage in my coronary artery was fixed, I still have other plaques that could rupture and cause a heart attack."

- "The book points out that my risks would be minimized if my blood pressure were under 115/75 and my LDL less than 80, and that statins, beta-blockers and ACE inhibitors are particularly effective."

- "Since these medicines are so safe, and can reduce my risks, is there any reason for me not to take them?"

Sometimes people may undergo a CAT scan to measure the amount of calcium deposited in the coronary arteries. (This is not a standard medical test but is becoming more widely available. Depending where you live, you may hear advertisements on the radio or even know someone who has had the test.) The general perception is that a low calcium score means there is no reason to worry and no reason for treatment. While a low score is better than a high score, even a zero score does not mean that you do not have small plaques that are capable of rupturing. Remember that the plaques that rupture tend to be the ones that are filled with fat, not the ones that have dense calcium in them, and the ruptured ones are those that trigger heart attacks, strokes and sudden death. This has been established by several studies. It is not an issue in doubt. Do not confuse low risk with no risk.

What to Do Now

Since you already know you have heart disease, the only kind of medical care you can afford to accept is optimal care. Whether you have coronary artery disease, abnormal cholesterol or high blood pressure, you are in a high-risk group, and you cannot afford to be passive. If you have cardiovascular disease and have not had a heart attack, but have a first-degree relative who has had a heart attack, angioplasty or bypass operation, the time to start with the program is when you are at least 10 years younger than the age of your relative when he or she was first diagnosed.

- Your blood pressure needs to be less than 115/75.
- Your LDL cholesterol level must be 80 or less if you have had a heart attack, an angioplasty or a bypass operation, or have been diagnosed with even mild to moderate coronary disease on an angiogram or cardiac catheterization (see Figures 8.1 and 8.3 in Chapter 8). If you have any other form of cardiovascular disease, your LDL should be less than 100.
- A beta-blocker will reduce your risk of sudden death if you have coronary disease, high blood pressure, or heart failure. Even if your blood pressure is less than 115/75, if you have any of these conditions you should be started on a low dose (with appropriate dosage adjustments later on).
- If you have diabetes, you need to have a doctor who insists on optimal glucose control. That means you are aiming for normal glucose and HgA_{1c}. Even if you can't get there, working toward

that goal is crucial. As a diabetic, your risk of a heart attack or dying young is about the same as someone who already has symptoms from coronary artery disease, so you need to follow the strictest components of this plan.

- If you smoke, quitting can be the most important thing you can do to stay alive, but it is also the hardest. Develop a plan with your doctor, but realize that the Before It Happens Plan works whether you quit now or 10 years from now.

- If you have siblings or children, tell them that they are at risk for heart disease and should visit their doctor and follow this plan in a way that is right for them. Your children should be evaluated at an age 10 years younger than the age at which you were first diagnosed.

These medicines—aspirin, statins, beta-blockers and ACE inhibitors—will reverse functional abnormalities of the cardiovascular system, stabilize and perhaps reverse at least some of the structural changes, and extend your life. They have also been proven to be safe. Despite the strength of their impact, they do not, however, cure you from coronary artery disease or cardiovascular disease in general. Fortunately, they are so effective that they will keep you alive long enough to see the benefits of emerging science, such as gene therapy, that may bring the true cure for cardiovascular disease. And at the very least, this plan will help you avoid a disabling heart attack or stroke, and will give you enough time to figure out how to improve your lifestyle.

The Reality of Heart Disease

If you already have heart disease, then it is vital that you be treated aggressively. Your numbers need to be optimal to assure that you stay alive.

- Your LDL needs to be < 80; your blood pressure needs to be < 115/75.

- Additional testing—a stress test, an echocardiogram, a CAT scan, etc.—is unnecessary. If you already have had symptoms of angina or have been diagnosed with high blood pressure or high cholesterol, you have heart disease.
- If you have diabetes, you need optimal glucose control.
- If you're a smoker, you need to quit.

Your doctor will choose a statin for your cholesterol, and consider ACE inhibitors, beta-blockers, and possibly a diuretic to keep your blood pressure down.

CHAPTER 10

If You Have Diabetes

SOME THINGS IN MEDICINE ARE PREDICTABLE. ONE IS THAT diabetics are well educated about their disease. Unfortunately, if you rely on your doctor, the American Diabetes Association or most other resources (books, magazines, the Internet etc.), you will not get the whole story.

As one example, you know that you need to control your glucose level, and that you are doing a good job when you get your HgA_{1c} down to 7 percent (the recommendation of the American Diabetes Association and the American Heart Association). You know that this will reduce your risk of cardiovascular disease, kidney disease and blindness.

However, most diabetics don't know that even if they achieve this level of control, they are still not optimally treated. Yes, your risk is lower when your HgA_{1c} is 7 percent instead of 8 or 9 percent, but getting your HgA_{1c} below 6 percent doesn't just lower your risk, it minimizes your risk.

The goal of 7 percent is a compromise between the benefits of tighter control and the small risk from your sugars going too low. If you suffer from frequent hypoglycemia (times when your sugar is too low), this is an appropriate compromise. Despite the concern about hypoglycemia, this is a problem that is unusual for most diabetics to have. When I lecture to other doctors, I frequently ask when the last time was that they took care of a diabetic. Any busy doctor takes care of several diabetics each day. Then I ask when the last time was that they had a patient with symptoms from low blood sugar. This question is followed by silence. I can see the doctors trying to remember— but they can't. The reason is that this is really uncommon. Yes, the likelihood of symptomatic hypoglycemia can be three times higher for someone with an HgA_{1c} under 7 than for someone with a level above 9, but with these infrequent episodes balanced against the benefits of tighter control, the lower target is definitely superior. In essence, your treatment is limited by fear of a problem that is unlikely to affect you. If you are unsure, ask your doctor these two questions.

- "Do you treat diabetics frequently?"
- "I am concerned about hypoglycemia. To get a sense of how common this problem is, when was the last time you took care of an adult-onset diabetic who suffered from symptomatic hypoglycemia?"

Practically speaking, the possibility that you may suffer from other side effects if you aim for better control of your sugars is a gross misperception. Multiple studies show that your risk of serious complications from diabetes is minimized with the tightest control possible, even with the potential for episodes of low blood sugar. Studies prove that a HgA_{1c} of 7 percent is not good enough, that your risk is even lower when your level becomes normal, less than 6 percent (see Figure 10.1).

You could check to see if your doctor knows this by asking what your HgA_{1c} should be in an optimal setting, but if you do, and your doctor doesn't know the data, the question will backfire. You would then need to explain the scientific evidence to your doctor to convince him or her that you know better. Do you think it will be easy to convince your doctor that you know more and then get him or her to admit it? That is what he or she would need to do in order to treat you according to the standards you seek. It isn't going to happen, so take a safer and more successful approach, such as the following:

- "I have a picture from a book that I would like you to look at because it explains to me why I need to improve my glucose control enough to lower my HgA_{1c} under 6 percent, if at all possible." (Show Figure 10.1.)

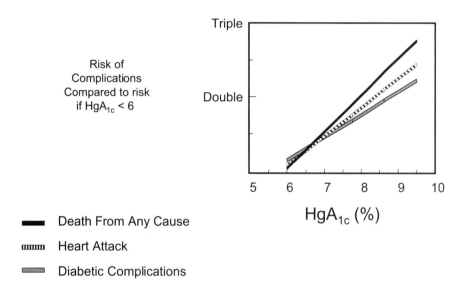

Diabetic Complications Increase Markedly with Even Small Increases in HgA₁c Level

Figure 10.1   Although the goal set by the American Diabetes Association (ADA) for HgA_{1c} is 7 percent, that is not the level at which your risk is minimized. Some diabetics, especially insulin-dependent diabetics, are prone to hypoglycemia, a potentially dangerous problem, so the ADA goal of 7 percent seems to be a reasonable compromise between the benefit of reducing risks of diabetes complications and decreasing the potential for hypoglycemia.

But if you are not at high risk of hypoglycemia, your overall health will be better if you strive to achieve an HgA_{1c} level of 6 percent or less—a normal level.

If you aren't sure whether it is worth it, consider your risks with an HgA_{1c} of 8 percent (this seems to be the typical level for many diabetics). Compared to getting under 6 percent, your risk of dying is nearly twice as high, your risk of a heart attack is more than 50 percent higher and of any major diabetes complication about 50 percent higher as well.

- "How can you adjust my medicines to achieve this goal, with the understanding that I will continue to work on tightening up my diet?"

The Plan for Diabetics

You have made a major step toward redefining your goals for glucose control with your doctor. Once you get to this point, you should feel good because you have taken control of your health plan in a way that will reduce your risk of complications from diabetes. But you know that these are tough goals to reach. You probably have struggled with your diet and have seen your HgA_{1c} hover well above 7 percent, and have wondered whether you can really get it down to 6 percent.

If your HgA_{1c} level is below 6 percent already, you may think that you have eliminated your risk from diabetes. Unfortunately, you are wrong; you remain at high risk. Your coronary arteries are as abnormal as someone who has already had a heart attack. In either case, since your goal is to stay alive and healthy, this plan is for you. Many diabetics don't know it, but the most powerful way to reduce your risk of a heart attack or stroke has little to do with your glucose control.

The two things that will reduce your risk the most are lowering your blood pressure and reducing your cholesterol.

You may be thinking that your blood pressure and cholesterol level are good enough, either because you are taking medicines already or because your doctor has told you that you don't need to. You may think your blood pressure is okay if it is as low as 130/80 and that your cholesterol is good enough if it is less than 200, since the standard guidelines say so. But the scientific studies say otherwise, with over-whelming evidence establishing that your risk of a heart attack, stroke and premature death can be further reduced dramatically with treat-ment. The standard guidelines mislead your doctor about your risks. Although the levels considered acceptable are *acceptable,* they are not *optimal,* and the recommendations in the guidelines leave your risk twice as high as it will be once you implement this plan.

That's right, this plan will cut your risk of a heart attack, stroke or premature death in half. There is no other plan that reduces your risk as much, no exercise program and no diet. But if you were to start exercising and dieting, the effects would add to the benefits of this

The Plan for People with Diabetes

- Your LDL needs to be < 80 using a statin.
- Your blood pressure needs to be < 115/75 (both numbers)
- You need an ACE inhibitor to protect your blood vessels and keep your plaques from rupturing.
- If you have an abnormal ECG or echocardiogram, you need to take a beta-blocker (if the abnormalities indicate a hypertrophied or weakened heart).
- You need to take an aspirin (81 mg) each day.
- You need your HDL > 40 (man) or > 50 (woman).
- You need your HgA_{1c} to be < 6%, unless you are prone to hypoglycemia.
- Recent studies indicate that when a diabetic needs a beta-blocker, carvedilol is better than the others.

plan, so they are worthwhile as well. But you know they are not so easy, so while you continue to try to improve your lifestyle, you can reduce your risk of heart attacks and strokes by starting with the Before It Happens Plan for diabetics now.

Diabetes and Your Cardiovascular System

Because you have diabetes, even without any other medical problem, you are 2 to 4 times as likely to suffer a heart attack and 2 to 4 times as likely to have a stroke as someone without diabetes. In 1999, according to the American Diabetes Association, 450,000 adult diabetics died, two-thirds (300,000) of whom died from cardiovascular disease.

You've read elsewhere in the book about the dangers of plaque developing in your blood vessels. In the absence of diabetes, the process starts in by your 20s and gets advanced by your 40s or 50s. As a diabetic, you will develop considerable plaque much earlier, starting in your teens and becoming widespread in your 20s. This rapid plaque

Are you a candidate for the Before It Happens Plan?

Andrea is 46 and diabetic. Her glucose control is ideal, even by my standards. She doesn't realize it, but her biggest risk is cardiovascular. Two-thirds of diabetics die from heart disease, but few take an ACE inhibitor or a statin. Using these two medicines would reduce Andrea's risk by more than a third.

development in diabetics comes from two causes: altered metabolism of proteins and fats as well as diabetes-related inflammation.

Excess sugar in the blood attaches to circulating proteins and fats, altering their function and structure. These larger molecules no longer flow freely through the circulation, making the blood thicker, in a way that promotes the formation of blood clots within the arteries. When cholesterol is glycosylated (the term used when glucose is attached), it gets trapped in the arterial walls, contributing to the growth of the plaques.

Diabetics either lack insulin or are resistant to its action. In either case, the loss of insulin's effects on the lining of the blood vessels allows any inflammation to go unchecked. So when the glycosylated cholesterol gets trapped and the immune system tries harder to digest and/or remove it, the body can't seem to limit the inflammation, and it escalates. The result is the development of inflamed and fat-filled plaques vulnerable to abrupt rupture.

For this reason, many have suggested that the newer insulin-sensitizing drugs, used for control of blood sugar, could also reduce the inflammation within the walls of the arteries and theoretically reduce your risk of a heart attack or stroke. This hypothesis is currently being tested in trials. Although we won't know for several years whether these medications will result in a reduction in cardiovascular risk, they are medicines I favor in my practice.

Damage to the peripheral arteries also occurs in diabetics and is cause for worry, causing pain or discomfort in the muscles of the legs with exercise. For many diabetics, the arterial disease develops in parallel with damage to the small nerves of the legs. The combination of peripheral artery disease with nerve damage that can come with diabetes is very dangerous. Typically not felt by the patient, small cuts or punctures can develop in the feet and can go unnoticed for weeks, often ulcerating, becoming infected, or refusing to heal. Extreme cases can become life threatening, even necessitating amputation of toes, feet or legs. Each year, 80,000 diabetics require an amputation.

The Guidelines Don't Take the Risk Seriously Enough

Perhaps you have read the recommendations by the American Diabetes Association. If so, you know that there is a lot of discussion about strategies to reduce your risk of heart attacks and strokes by more rigorous control of your blood pressure and cholesterol Unfortunately, the ADA stops short of recommending anything, despite overwhelming evidence.

The recommendations by the American Diabetes Association include a blood pressure of less than 130/70, an LDL less than 100 and initiation of aspirin therapy at the age of 40. Your risk is not minimized with this strategy, but it is if you set your targets for blood pressure less than 115/75, LDL less than 80, and HgA_{1c} under 6 percent, in addition to taking low-dose aspirin therapy.

I can assure you that the doctors I know are implementing these approaches for themselves, and you will want to also, once you see the proof.

Control of Blood Pressure

There is no controversy about the fact that lowering your blood pressure reduces your risk of heart attacks and strokes, and every medical group agrees that tight blood pressure control is more important in diabetics than in the general population. That's why the current guidelines from the American Diabetes Association and the Joint National Commission (the blood pressure guidelines committee, referred to as JNC) recommend that your blood pressure should be 130/80 or less in contrast to the recommendation of 140/90 or less in people without diabetes.

But this target (130/80) is a compromise made in the interest of the cost to society, not one selected in your best interest. If you look at the most recent guidelines*, you will see that scientific studies prove that your risk is minimized when your blood pressure is less than 115/75 (based on studies from the 1960s up to 2003). The reason that they recommend that your blood pressure be reduced to less than 130/80, instead of 115/75, is their concern for the cost to society of the more aggressive target. It is just too expensive to treat over 100 million Americans aggressively enough to get their blood pressure to 115/75.

When your life is at stake, you can't afford to compromise.

The specifics of blood pressure control can follow several paths. Most guidelines refer to ACE inhibitors, beta-blockers and diuretics in one order or another. Another kind of medicine that is frequently used is a calcium channel blocker. Calcium blockers are useful drugs, but review of the hundreds of studies using them suggests that the benefits may not be as consistent, and that they may even increase the risk in some people. In light of the inconsistency in the data, I believe calcium blockers should be used only when the other medications in this plan fail to control blood pressure, as I discuss in Chapter 7.

Work with your doctor—each person's blood pressure will be responsive to different medication, and the process of controlling your blood pressure should occur slowly to minimize side effects. Bringing down blood pressure too quickly can leave you feeling tired and sometimes dizzy. Since most patients require more than one agent, I gauge which one to use first on an individual basis. Since ACE inhibitors and beta-blockers not only reduce blood pressure, but also protect the blood vessels and stabilize plaques, they are my first choic-

*Available at http://www.nhlbi.nih.gov/guidelines/hypertension/express.pdf, page 15.

es. Diuretics (water pills) are beneficial in that they lower blood pressure, but they are my second choice since they do not directly improve vascular health.

Many doctors consider beta-blockers undesirable for diabetics. The reason that would appear justified is that beta-blockers can reduce the symptoms you would experience when your blood sugar is low. Unless low blood sugar is happening to you a lot, the advantages of blood pressure lowering are likely to outweigh that risk. The other reason cited is that beta-blockers can worsen glucose control. This is true for most beta-blockers, but not true for the beta-blocker carvedilol, so it is the preferred beta-blocker for diabetics.

An additional advantage of ACE inhibitors is that they can favorably affect glucose utilization and insulin sensitivity, which means glucose control improves and HgA_{1c} levels drop (a little, but a little is good). The beta-blocker carvedilol is similar to ACE inhibitors in that it can improve HgA_{1c} and prevent the development of diabetes in people at risk. Other beta-blockers tend to have the opposite effect, making carvedilol the preferred beta-blocker for diabetics and those at risk for developing diabetes.

You need to ask your doctor specifically to prescribe an ACE inhibitor.

Usually, doctors use ACE inhibitors only if you have high blood pressure or heart failure (that is when your heart is weak). When you realize that your coronary arteries look the same as those of someone who has already had a heart attack, it's not hard to realize that an ACE inhibitor could make a big difference for diabetics and others with vascular disease. The HOPE trial evaluated whether ACE inhibitors could do more. Over 9,000 patients were treated for over 4 years with either the ACE inhibitor ramipril or placebo. The HOPE trial proved that the ACE inhibitor ramipril reduced the risk of heart attacks, strokes and premature deaths for diabetics who had normal blood pressure.

The data are clear: high blood pressure is a bigger risk for you than it is for a person without diabetes, and lowering your pressure under 115/75, or at least 20 points lower than it currently is, will cut your risk in half. If you are paying attention to what this plan promises, you should start to realize that my promise, to cut your risk in half, is actually an understatement. Just reducing blood pressure gets your risk 50 percent lower, and added to that are the benefits of aspirin and cholesterol management, to reduce your risk further.

Control of Cholesterol

The mandate to treat abnormalities of cholesterol is quite clear. Notice I did not say to treat elevations of cholesterol, but rather, to treat abnormalities. The blood test you take to measure your cholesterol levels is only an approximation of the real problem, the cholesterol in the walls of your arteries.

The standard guidelines recommend treating you (as a diabetic) as if your coronary arteries are as bad as someone who has already had a heart attack. That is justified by many scientific studies. Unfortunately, those guidelines do not recommend treatment to a level that would minimize your risk, choosing only to partially reduce it.

The Before It Happens Plan relies on the best data available to establish a target significantly lower, thereby reducing risk 20 to 30 percent lower.

Many other doctors have proposed such strict control of cholesterol in diabetics. A recent study showed that diabetics treated with the statin simvastatin were at a 20 to 25 percent lower risk of heart attacks, strokes and premature deaths. Those investigators recommended that any diabetic with a total cholesterol above 135 (meaning many had a bad cholesterol, the LDL, as low as 80) should automatically receive a statin. I've discussed this plan with other doctors, and recently I've been asked why I "only" recommend reducing LDL below 80, instead of 60 or 70. I believe the studies underway will prove that 60 or 70 is best, but right now the best data available say that 80 is optimal. Keep asking your doctor, or visit my website at http://beforeithappens.com to learn when new data push these targets even lower.

One of the most important studies defining the role of statins for diabetics is the Heart Protection Study. In this study, over 6,000 diabetics with a total cholesterol level of at least 135 mg/dl, but not high enough to warrant treatment, were randomly chosen to receive the statin simvastatin or a placebo. Simvastatin markedly reduced the risk of heart attacks and death even in those diabetics who started with an LDL around 100 or lower. By the end of the study, the statin reduced LDL cholesterol level under 80, with no evidence of increased side effects (this is shown in Chapter 4). The CARDS study confirmed this important benefit using atorvastatin.

As a diabetic, based on this and other studies, you need to have an LDL under 80, and you should be treated with a statin to do so.

An important consideration when seeking optimal care is the management of triglyceride levels (another form of cholesterol that is only minimally improved with a statin). Your triglyceride level is not as important as LDL level in your predicting risk, but it is still important. If your triglyceride levels are high in conjunction with a reduced HDL level, your risk is increased, and you do need to address this issue as well. However, the medications used for management of triglycerides are not as simple or safe as those advocated as the primary components of the Before It Happens Plan, and, especially if you are also taking a statin, you should be seen by a physician experienced in the treatment of diabetics with hypertriglyceridemia. This will ensure that the therapy can be utilized safely and effectively.

Too frequently, patients don't benefit from scientific evidence.

Despite the compelling evidence supporting this plan, many people still are not being treated optimally. Sophia, a 47-year-old diabetic and a close friend, is one. Diagnosed three years ago, she has been treated with oral hypoglycemic agents and her HgA_{1c} is 6.1 percent. She thinks that she is doing well since her glucose control is better than the American Diabetes Association recommendations. Sophia did not know her blood pressure or her cholesterol level but was under the impression they were "fine." Even if they were, I told her, the HOPE trial proved she should be treated with an ACE inhibitor. Another study, the Heart Protection Study, tells us that she should be strongly considered for statin therapy.

What the Hope Trial and the Heart Protection Study Mean for Sophia—and You

In the HOPE trial, the ACE inhibitor ramipril was given randomly to half of the people in the study. The primary goal was to assess the impact on those who were at high risk but had no evidence of high blood pressure or heart failure, two places where it was already established that an ACE inhibitor is proven to be effective. The population studied were people 55 and older who had diabetes as well as either another cardiovascular risk factor (hypertension, increased cholesterol, positive family history, cigarette smoking) or established vascular disease (history of heart attack, stroke, or peripheral arterial disease). After four and one-half years of treatment, it was clear that the ACE inhibitor therapy reduced the risk of heart attacks, strokes, heart failure, and death.

The Heart Protection Study involved over 20,000 people with known diabetes or vascular disease who did not require statin therapy based on the standard guidelines. They were randomly chosen to receive simvastatin (a statin) or placebo. The effect of simvastatin on diabetics was remarkable, reducing the risk of heart disease by about 25 percent, protecting even those whose LDL cholesterol levels were less than 116 mg/dl at the start of the study. (This group also had a risk 25 percent lower.)

- "I understand how important it is to control my sugars and I am doing the best I can. I also understand that controlling my cholesterol and blood pressure will reduce my risk of a heart attack, stroke or kidney failure."

- "Why shouldn't I be treated with a statin like in the Heart Protection Study and the CARDS Study, and an ACE inhibitor as in the HOPE trial?"
- "Since JNC-7 guidelines point out that having my blood pressure under 115/75 minimizes my risk, and this book I am reading says that getting my LDL below 80 would also, shouldn't these be our goals?"

Sophia is not yet 55 and at first review, it did not appear she was exactly like the patients in the HOPE trial because even though she had diabetes, she would only have been eligible for the study if she had another risk factor. However, I knew she had significant coronary disease based on other information available about heart disease: A study at the Cleveland Clinic ascertained that 60 percent of people over 40 have significant plaques, as do more than 85 percent of those over 50. Since other studies have shown that diabetes brings out coronary disease significantly earlier in life, Sophia, in her 40s, almost certainly had arteries that looked like she was in her 50s.

For these reasons, I wanted Sophia on the following medicines:

1. An ACE inhibitor: ACE inhibitors block several chemical processes that lead to plaque rupture. In experimental models, ACE inhibitors can also reduce the fat content of plaques. These effects would enhance the stability of plaques, which would explain the findings in the HOPE trial that the ACE inhibitors reduce the risk of heart attack, stroke and early death.
2. A statin: Statins reduce cholesterol levels and stabilize plaques as well. ACE inhibitors and statins also reduce the damage caused if a plaque were to rupture. This explains the findings in the Heart Protection Study regarding the reduction in heart attacks, strokes and premature deaths.

Unfortunately, Sophia's general practitioner had told Sophia that an ACE inhibitor was not relevant to her. I was surprised by this response. Despite the fact that the diabetes guidelines were updated as recently as 2002 and 2003, they omitted any recommendations based on HOPE and the Heart Protection Study. The guidelines concentrated intensely on tight glucose control and recommend "tight control" of blood pressure and cholesterol using targets that are too high, in effect making their idea of "tight control" far from optimal.

It seems as though the diabetes specialists are too worried about stepping into the domain of the cardiologists, while most cardiologists defer to the diabetes doctors to make the diabetes recommendations. Neither seems to be paying attention to the studies—even studies approved by the FDA such as HOPE and the Heart Protection Study. The political forces are impeding the dissemination of these lifesaving studies to practicing physicians and patients.

Perhaps the main reason why such aggressive strategies are not recommended is made clear by reading the standard guidelines. Consistently, the standard guidelines acknowledge that the impact of the therapies is impressive, but also point out that it is not cost-effective to apply these treatments as broadly as the scientific data support. Your doctor probably has not read these passages in the guidelines, but they are stated explicitly. For example, the National Cholesterol Education Panel, Adult Treatment Plan-III explicitly stated that despite the benefits to you, treating thousands or millions of people like you would be too costly to recommend.

Is this how you want your treatment to be determined? Neither did Sophia. She made an appointment with her endocrinologist to get started on an ACE inhibitor and a statin.

Although tighter glucose control has been shown to reduce the risk of kidney failure and other microvascular diseases, you need to know that your risk of heart attacks, strokes and premature death remains high. I want you to focus on glucose control and also get your blood pressure and cholesterol to optimal levels using ACE inhibitors and statins in particular. When beta-blocker therapy is indicated, the effects on glucose control may dictate selection of carvedilol. Low-dose aspirin can further reduce morbidity and mortality. Together the medicines in the plan improve quality of life, and keep you around longer to enjoy it.

The Reality of Diabetes

- Sugar control is only the first step for a diabetic. To stay alive you need to protect your vasculature. Unfortunately, many doctors are not aware of the importance of vascular protection.

- Many doctors don't realize how much lower your risk will be with lower blood pressure and cholesterol levels.

- Be assertive and committed. The Before It Happens treatments can save your life. Your new knowledge gives you the power to control your health and well-being. Once you convince your doctor to treat you according to this plan, you have planted the seed for subsequent patients to be viewed as candidates as well, meaning you will become the first of many whose lives will be saved.

CHAPTER 11

If You Are Overweight (Even 10 Pounds)

IT'S TOUGH TO LOSE WEIGHT, ISN'T IT? AREN'T YOU TIRED OF hearing about the health risks of the extra weight and the benefits of losing even 10 or 15 pounds?

I have something more important to discuss with you. I don't
want you to feel frustrated and
stressed. I want you to reduce your

> Relax about your weight for a little while. (Did you ever think you'd hear a doctor say that?)

risk of heart disease by 50 percent or more, whether or not you can lose your excess weight. You can actually derive more benefit for your health following the Before It Happens Plan than you could with weight loss alone. Best of all, when you are finally able to lose the extra weight, that will add to the benefits of this plan.

The purpose of this chapter is to explain the easy parts of this plan; those tasks you can actually accomplish now, as opposed to Chapters 17 and 18, which discuss the harder stuff, how to actually lose weight. Whether you're at midlife or older, the presence of even 10 or 15 pounds may increase your risk of suffering a heart attack or stroke, or dying from cardiovascular disease or cancer (see Figure 11.1). This chapter provides a plan for you whether you are 10 to 15 pounds over-weight or morbidly obese. The more overweight you feel, the more important it is to implement this plan, but in any case, the plan will reduce your risk.

As you know, the plan is based on the use of safe prescription med-ications that will help prevent or control heart disease. However, after

Your Risks from Cardiovascular Disease
Are Increased Even If You Are Only a Little Overweight

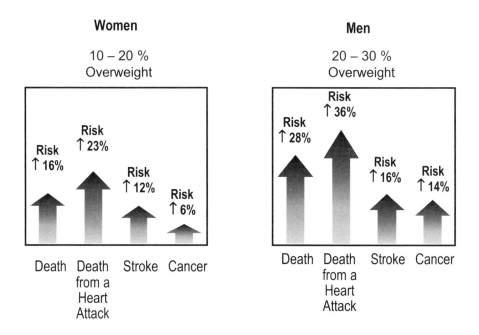

Figure 11.1 Everyone knows that obesity increases risks. Most doctors talk about an important link between being overweight and getting cancer. But the scientific evidence shows that being even mildly overweight puts you at higher risk of dying from a heart attack or suffering a stroke than of cancer.

If you are a woman whose ideal weight is 130, and you weigh 145, your risk of dying from a heart attack is 23 percent higher because of those extra 10 to 15 pounds. Same story for a man whose ideal weight is 180 and weighs 205.

Those extra pounds are more than a cosmetic issue.

the bad press concerning several of the drugs given for weight loss, you may be understandably wary of the thought of signing on for other prescription medications. I can assure you that safety is of paramount importance to me, and the drugs used in this plan are selected because of their effectiveness and their outstanding safety record in millions of people over decades of use.

Why You Need to Do This Now

In the 1930s, several life insurance companies evaluated how excess weight affected their prospective policy holders' risks of dying young. The data showed convincingly that it was necessary and justified to charge higher premiums for people who were overweight—not just those who were obese. This conclusion was corroborated by many later studies that established the relationship between excess weight and the risk of suffering a heart attack or dying young.

Again and again, as studies addressed the same issues over the following decades, the same relationship was shown—that increased weight increases the risk of cardiovascular death. In the 1950s an American Cancer Society study revealed that men who are 10 to 20 percent above ideal body weight have a 15 percent higher risk of death, while women whose weight is 10 to 20 percent above ideal body weight have a 17 percent risk of premature death. Although the American Cancer Society study had intended to learn how excess weight related to cancer, most notable was the finding that the excess weight primarily increased risk of cardiovascular death, *not* cancer. Those 10 to 20 percent above ideal body weight were 23 percent more likely to die young from cardiovascular disease (same risk for men and women), and also had a higher risk of dying from a stroke.

In the early 1990s, the Harvard Alumni Study showed that even if you were at the upper end of the range for normal weight, your risk would be higher than someone at the low end of the normal range. This finding was confirmed in a study that was limited to women.

In all of these studies, the degree to which people were overweight correlated closely with the amount of the increase in risk of premature cardiovascular death. These observations get pretty scary for those of us who think we are relatively safe because we only need to lose about 10 pounds.

The Plan for Overweight or Obese People
....

- Your blood pressure needs to be < 115/75.
- Your LDL needs to be < 100, or < 80 if you need aggressive protection.*
- Your HDL needs to be > 40 (man) or > 50 (woman).
- If you are over 50 you need to take aspirin (81 mg) each day; start at 40 years old if you need aggressive protection.*
- Protect your vasculature with an ACE inhibitor if you need aggressive protection.*
- Reduce your risk of sudden death with a beta-blocker if you need aggressive protection.*
- Your HgA_{1c} needs to be < 6%; get checked even if no one has told you that you have diabetes.

* Aggressive protection is needed for those with a BMI > 30, diabetics, smokers, people with a history of a heart attack or stroke, those with a first-degree relative with coronary artery disease or sudden death (sibling, parent, or child) and those with evidence of hypertrophy or weakening of the heart on ECG or echocardiogram.

Excess Weight Causes Other Problems

People who are overweight more frequently have diabetes, hypertension and high cholesterol. In addition, many people who are even mildly overweight have associated borderline diabetes, borderline blood pressure or slightly increased cholesterol levels. In each case, treatment of these coexisting conditions to achieve optimal status will lower risk.

Borderline diabetes (also referred to as diet-controlled diabetes), high-normal blood pressure (between 115/75 and 140/90) and LDL cholesterol level above 100 each increases your risk of cardiovascular disease. Considering that your likelihood of having fatty deposits in your arteries is markedly increased as your weight increases, any of these additional problems would make your risk scary. On the positive side, this plan can reverse each of these processes.

What Happens to Your Vascular System When You Are Overweight?

Excess weight accelerates the development of atherosclerosis (presence of fatty plaques in the walls of your arteries). The National Institutes of Health's study, the Pathobiological Determinants of Atherosclerosis in Youth (PDAY), confirmed studies that proved that the plaques start when you are 20 to 30 years old, and showed that the process starts earlier and the plaques become more widespread in people who are overweight. The risk increases even for those only 10 to 15 percent overweight.

The development of these plaques in your arteries is well understood (see Chapter 2). The problems start with cholesterol deposits in the walls of your arteries, and as your body tries to compensate and stabilize these plaques, the activation of the immune system to help with this repair process also paradoxically increases the vulnerability of these plaques to rupture. (The plaques that are the most likely to rupture are the smaller ones, which do not cause symptoms and are undetectable by any of our standard tests.) If you have a plaque that ruptures, a blood clot forms, blocking blood flow in that artery and causing a heart attack or sudden death.

Are you a candidate for the Before It Happens Plan?

Tom is 63 years old and 70 pounds overweight. His HDL (the good cholesterol) is quite high, so he thinks he has nothing to worry about. But Tom's LDL is high too. His risk is 1 in 166 that he will have a heart attack or stroke despite his HDL. According to this plan, he should be taking an aspirin, a statin and an ACE inhibitor. Together, these would reduce his risk by 50 percent.

This process is even more aggressive in teenagers who are overweight, with the likelihood of plaques forming by your mid-20s nearly double if you are very overweight. Is it possible that these plaques go away if you lose the weight? I am sure it is possible, but there are no data that prove it to be so. Therefore, even if you were only overweight for a few years as a kid or teen, you probably had plaques build up that are almost certainly still there. Even if you have been carrying the extra weight for only five or ten years, you still need this plan, because your blood vessels have already suffered. Since the medicines in the Before It Happens Plan are so safe, you need to be treated more aggressively.

Assessing Your Personal Risk

Assessing the amount of excess body fat and its distribution are powerful ways to predict your risk. The tendency of fat to deposit in the central trunk of the body (around the abdomen) more than in the peripheral area (including the buttocks and thighs), is a marker for metabolic abnormalities that are similar to those of diabetes, and leads to some of the same risks of developing more serious heart disease. When fat is deposited predominantly in the central trunk along with various combinations of high cholesterol, high triglyceride levels, high blood pressure or diabetes (or insulin resistance), it is called the metabolic syndrome. People with the metabolic syndrome are at significantly increased risk of cardiovascular disease. Even the conventional guidelines recommend intensive therapy for people with metabolic syndrome.

I disagree with the standard guidelines because the average risk for the general population is not what should determine your care. The only thing that matters about your care is your risk. The standard targets for blood pressure and cholesterol are not good enough for you. The Before It Happens Plan decreases your risks by defining targets that are optimal; targets that all agree are associated with the lowest possible risk, using old medicines that have been studied extensively and used by millions of people for decades. These approaches are safe and are based on scientific proof.

One way to assess your risk is a measure called the waist-to-hip ratio. Measure your waist just above your belly button and your hips at the point where your buttocks protrude the most, and divide your waist by your hip measurement. The higher your ratio is, the more likely you are to develop diabetes (especially if the ratio is greater than 0.95 for a man or 0.85 for a woman). Another simple way to approximate your risk is to measure your waist. If your waist is more than 40 inches (men) or 35 inches (women), you need this plan even more than you may think.

The most accurate way to quantify your risk is by calculating your body mass index, or BMI. BMI is equal to your weight (in kilograms) divided by your height (in meters) squared. Of course, you probably don't know your height in meters or how many kilograms you weigh, so you can use this version of the formula instead. BMI is equal to your weight (in pounds) divided by your height (in inches) squared, all multiplied by 703. If your BMI is above 25 you are overweight and if it is above 30 you are obese.

$$BMI = weight (pounds)/[height (inches)]^2 \times 703$$

The Plan for Overweight and Obese People

The Before It Happens Plan protects your blood vessels and reverses their functional and structural abnormalities.

Reduce LDL cholesterol levels. Even if you have no evidence of coronary artery disease, your LDL should be less than 100. If you are obese (body mass index > 30), have diabetes or have been diagnosed with coronary artery disease, are a smoker, have a first-degree relative with heart disease, or have a thickened or weak heart, your LDL should be under 80. Statins are powerful tools that will help you achieve this target.

Achieve optimal blood pressure levels. This should be defined as a level < 115/75 (or at least reduce your systolic blood pressure by at least 20 points). You should start with an ACE inhibitor. However, my strategy for selecting an additional medication, should it be required,

depends upon whether you are actively losing weight, since moderate-
or high-dose beta-blocker therapy can reduce your metabolic rate
(making it tougher to lose weight).

In such a case the second step should utilize a diuretic instead of a
beta-blocker. If your blood pressure remains above 115/75 after use
of an ACE inhibitor and a diuretic, the angiotensin receptor blocker
candesartan or the calcium blocker amlodipine are effective and have
been studied extensively, assuring their safety. I cannot say the same
for other calcium blockers. If your blood pressure were extreme,
above 150/100, then even if you are trying to lose weight, I would use
beta-blocker therapy as well.

If you are not actively losing weight (and you need to be honest with
yourself here), a beta-blocker would be the recommendation after an
ACE inhibitor and a diuretic, rather than candesartan or amlodipine.

Protect your vascular system with aspirin (after discussing it with
your doctor). Aspirin should be utilized at a dose of 81 mg once
daily if you are over 50 or post-menopausal, as long as your blood
pressure is satisfactory. Studies have shown that the risks of bleeding with aspirin are lower when you take a lower dose (81 mg, not
325 mg) and when your blood pressure is controlled. Risks can
increase when systolic blood pressure is above 180, so try to get your
pressure down to at least the 140s before starting the aspirin. If your
BMI is greater than 30, aspirin therapy should be started in your 40s.
If you are diabetic and your BMI is greater than 30, aspirin should
be started in your 30s. If you have any signs or a history of vascular
disease, or have a history of heart attacks, strokes or high blood
pressure in your family, then you should start in your 30s.

Whether you are obese or merely 10 to 15 pounds overweight, if
your blood pressure is less than 115/75 and your LDL is less than 100,
your doctor may tell you that you don't need to worry. Even in that
case, if you are 50 or post-menopausal or your BMI is above 30, you
should ask your doctor about low-dose aspirin therapy. Even low-dose
ACE inhibitor and statin therapies can reduce your risk further. ACE

inhibitors reduce risk in people with vascular disease, even if they don't have high blood pressure. The more overweight you are, the higher your risk and the more likely you are to benefit from an ACE inhibitor, even in the absence of high blood pressure. Ask your doctor whether it makes sense for you.

If you are overweight and just can't seem to lose the last 10 to 20 pounds, or you can, but can't keep it off, ask questions such as these:

- "I realize that my risk of heart disease is increased because I am overweight, and I am trying to lose the extra 10 to 20 pounds [or whatever amount is relevant for you]."
- "By middle age, I am likely to have coronary artery disease anyway, so with the added risk of being even 10 to 20 percent overweight, it makes sense to me to be treated more aggressively."
- "Even though I am not eager to take medicines, I understand that my risk of a heart attack or stroke is lowest if my blood pressure is under 115/75 and my LDL under 100."
- "Would I be a candidate for blood pressure medicines like beta-blockers and ACE inhibitors, as well as a statin for my cholesterol?"

For those of you who are obese, with a BMI above 30, these questions focus on your increased risk:

- "I realize I don't have high blood pressure, diabetes or very high cholesterol, but since my BMI is above 30, I realize that studies show that I am likely to have pretty extensive plaques forming in my coronary arteries, even if they aren't big enough to block blood flow."
- "Wouldn't this make me almost the type of patient studied in HOPE and the Heart Protection Study, and therefore someone whose risk could be reduced by an ACE inhibitor and a statin?"

The truth is, you would benefit, so make sure you ask the question firmly (but deferentially) in order to force the issue with your doctor.

What about the Excess Weight?

Eventually you ought to work on losing the excess weight. You'll like how you look, and you'll like how you feel. Unfortunately there is no magic for weight management.

Much is known about weight gain and obesity, but unfortunately little definitive information exists about how to take the weight off again. Several possible mechanisms focus on brain function, behavior and metabolism, but no therapy has been shown to be safe and effective at reversing the problem. For my opinion on the best way to diet, please refer to Chapter 18. In this chapter, I want to address the weight loss treatments that have been on the market recently.

Several agents have been developed and marketed, including prescription medications and those available over-the-counter. Some approaches are clearly dangerous and should not be considered at all. You may remember the fen-phen debacle, in which a combination of these two medicines turned out to be associated with the development of heart disease. Many are aware of the controversy surrounding ephedra-based over-the-counter dietary supplements, but many are not aware that there are reports in the literature that ephedra increases the risk of arrhythmias and death, and enough data to convince many that ephedra should be withdrawn from the market. Trying to lose 10 pounds, 20 pounds, or even 50 pounds is not worth it if these are your choices. Recently released products use a substance related to ephedra, but without the bad publicity, called synphedrine. Synphedrine may be just as bad, so it, too, should be avoided.

Subitramine and orlistat are prescription medicines that help many to lose weight, but they do have side effects that can be of concern, or at a minimum aggravating (subitramine can cause hypertension and increase cardiovascular risk; orlistat can cause diarrhea and intestinal discomfort). Neither of these drugs eliminates the problem that led to your weight gain in the first place, so even though you would lose weight taking them, what do you expect will happen after you stop?

Because neither subitramine nor orlistat has been used continuously for years in thousands of patients, let alone millions, we do not know with sufficient confidence that they are safe to continue to take long-term. Therefore I do not routinely recommend them. In more extreme cases, your doctor could recommend these medicines based on the balance between risks and benefits for you. There clearly are people who need these medications.

Several over-the-counter agents sold as dietary supplements are used widely. Billions of dollars are spent each year on dietary supplements, but none of these products has been studied nearly enough to make anyone confident that they are proven safe, let alone effective. So while many make sense, and I believe that many are likely to be safe and helpful, the scientific evidence does not exist to support their use, and certainly any claims pale compared to the scientific proof that exists for the components of this plan.

Scientifically there is no doubt that the prescription medicines recommended in this plan are safer than the prescription medicines or the over-the-counter agents available to help you lose weight. In addition, the medications in this plan are proven to reduce the risk of heart attacks, strokes and premature death.

So why take a chance when you can take control and decrease your risk?

The Reality of Being Overweight

- Excess weight, even only 10 pounds, greatly increases your risk of diabetes and heart disease. (And being diabetic leads to an even greater risk of heart disease.)
- You can reduce your risk of heart attacks and strokes 50 percent or more by paying attention to your heart health, even if you can't yet lose the extra weight.
- Your LDL needs to be < 100; your blood pressure needs to be < 115/75.

- Your doctor will choose a statin for your cholesterol, and consider ACE inhibitors, beta-blockers, and possibly a diuretic to keep your blood pressure down.

- With your doctor's okay, you should also take an aspirin (81 mg) each day to protect your vascular system.

- Your HgA_{1c} needs to be checked regularly to be certain you do not begin to show signs of diabetes.

CHAPTER 12

If You Smoke

WHEN YOU LIGHT UP A CIGARETTE IN FRONT OF A NON-SMOKER, especially a friend or family member, you know what they are thinking, and it's quite a relief when they don't say it. No one needs to be reminded about a bad habit over and again. Besides, they can't possibly understand how hard it is to quit, can they?

It isn't much better when you visit the doctor. If your doctor doesn't smoke, he or she probably looks at you with disbelief, wondering why you wouldn't want to quit. Of course you want to quit; it just isn't so easy.

Time after time, from one person after another, you hear the same thing and see the same reactions. Eventually, you can't help but feel a little guilty. Anyone with an addiction (and tobacco is an addiction) feels powerless, unable to stop their self-destructive behavior.

All anyone wants is to prevent you from dying young, and a major way to do that is prevent heart attacks and strokes. I know that the standard recommendations do not work for most smokers, and since you are still smoking, they do not work for you.

The Before It Happens Plan takes a different approach from any other, because I know how to reduce your risk of a heart attack or stroke whether or not you can quit. If you can quit, you'll be a lot better off, because your risk will be reduced even more. But you can cut your risk in half immediately by implementing this plan. I want you to take protective measures against heart disease immediately; then we can talk about how you really ought to quit smoking. In contrast to the standard smoking cessation strategies, this plan can be implemented successfully now, without requiring you to change your

---

The Plan for Smokers

- Your LDL needs to be < 80 using a statin.
- Your blood pressure needs to be < 115/75 (both numbers)
- You need an ACE inhibitor to protect your blood vessels and keep plaques from rupturing, even if you don't have high blood pressure.
- You need a beta-blocker if an ECG or echocardiogram suggests hypertrophy or weakness of your heart muscle.
- You need to take an aspirin (81 mg) each day.
- You need your HDL > 40 (man) or > 50 (woman).
- Your HgA_{1c} needs to be < 6%; get checked even if no one has told you that you have diabetes.

---

habits, control your urges, or damage your emotional well-being, all while reducing your risk of heart disease by 50 percent or more.

The plan will do for you what no other plan can   it will extend your life even if you can't quit. Before you quit, while you're trying to quit, and even after you quit, this plan will work for you.

The Effects of Smoking on the Blood Vessels

The effects of smoking have been studied extensively, so I can tell you with absolute certainty that you have a lot more damage in your heart and blood vessels than you think you do. Studies dating back to the 1950s have demonstrated rapid development of vascular disease in smokers. (The same holds true for people with diabetes, high blood pressure or high cholesterol, and each of these factors adds to the damage caused by smoking.) In a smoker, the fatty plaques that begin developing in the walls of the arteries in our 20s or 30s develop more rapidly and cause functional impairments of the blood vessels earlier in life.

Are you a candidate for the Before It Happens Plan?
••

Margaret is 55 but doesn't look it. She's careful about what she eats, takes care of herself and dresses well. For her, life seems good, except that she smokes, which means that her wonderful appearance is literally skin deep. Smoking has ravaged her blood vessels. By following this plan and taking an aspirin, a statin and an ACE inhibitor, Margaret's risk would be cut by 50 percent.

Smoking also makes your plaques unstable, increasing the likelihood of rupture (without warning) or of developing microscopic erosions on their surfaces. Ruptures and erosions both trigger the formation of blood clots, which block flow in the artery, leading to a heart attack, stroke or sudden death.

A study sponsored by the National Institutes of Health, called the Pathobiological Determinants of Atherosclerosis in Youth (PDAY), discovered that even smoking for a few years caused major damage to the blood vessels. Think about that; smoking as a teen or young adult for only a few years markedly accelerates the deposit of fat into the walls of the arteries, leaving you with more widespread and severe cardiovascular disease. If the damage begins as soon as you start smoking, imagine how your arteries look after smoking even a half a pack a day from young adulthood into midlife. PDAY revealed that almost 30 percent of people dying in their early 20s already had significant plaques in the arteries of their heart. The likelihood of having fat-filled vulnerable plaques was a shocking 44 percent higher in smokers.

While standard diagnostic tests will eventually pick up the narrowing in the arteries caused by calcium deposits and the plaques that have gotten big, neither of these kinds of plaques are the ones likely to rupture and cause a heart attack. At this point, there are no simple tests available to detect the smaller, cholesterol-filled plaques that are the high-risk lesions, vulnerable to rupture and more likely to cause a heart attack or sudden death. Despite the radio advertisements touting the power of high-tech CAT scans or the perception that stress tests are useful screening tests, neither can detect the plaques that put your life at risk. If you are a smoker, you have these vulnerable plaques. The good news is that the vulnerability can be reversed with the treatments of this plan.

Because smoking leads to changes in the structure and function of the cardiovascular system in a manner that markedly increases your risk, you need treatments that accomplish the following:

1. Stabilization of the vulnerable plaques

2. Restoration of the normal function of your cardiovascular system

3. Reversal of the structural changes that have been developing over the years of smoking and living the typical American lifestyle

A wealth of scientific data supports the combination of aspirin, statins, beta-blockers and ACE inhibitors to reduce the fat content in the walls of the arteries, decrease the inflammation, and strengthen the thin layers covering the plaques.

Insist on Optimal Protection for Your Heart and Vasculature

• Statins reduce the fat deposits in your plaques, reduce the likelihood of rupture and improving vessel function.

• ACE inhibitors improve vascular function and enhance plaque stability.

• Beta-blockers prevent heart arrhythmias and reduce the risk of sudden death in people with coronary artery disease (especially in people with a history of a heart attack), high blood pressure and heart failure.

You Need Optimal, Not Average, Treatment

As a smoker, you have damage to your blood vessels that is about the same as in a diabetic. That means you should be treated as aggressively as a person whose coronary artery disease is bad enough to have caused a heart attack.

In theory, if you already have high blood pressure or high cholesterol, or if you already have suffered a heart attack, then your doctor should have known to treat you similarly to the steps of this plan.

But remember the point I've stressed throughout: Your treatment must be optimal, especially for you as a smoker. Don't let your doctor convince you to be happy with the target levels published by professional societies and government agencies. These guidelines are not strict enough.

If your doctor treats you to keep your blood pressure at the standard goal, 135/80, you still have twice the risk of a heart attack, stroke or death from cardiovascular disease over the next decade than a similar person with a blood pressure less than 115/75. If your LDL is 110, your risk is 25 to 30 percent higher than if it were under 80. An ACE inhibitor protects your vasculature so that even if you have optimal blood pressure, it reduces your risk more than 20 percent. These medicines are safer than vitamins, and in contrast to vitamins, they are proven to work.

Your doctor may tell you that your risk is low enough even if you don't achieve the targets of the Before It Happens Plan. It's true that your risks are low, but you need to be ready to tell your doctor that you want your risks minimized, not merely reduced, as described in this plan.

- "I know I will be a lot healthier when I quit smoking, but I also know that I will still be at higher risk of heart attacks and strokes than a nonsmoker for several years after I quit, not to mention my higher risk right now."

- "Since smoking causes my arteries to look like the arteries of someone with advanced diabetes or even a person who has had a heart attack already, I know that I need to be treated just as aggressively as they are."
- "Therefore, can you tell me how we can lower my LDL-cholesterol under 80 and my blood pressure under 115/75?"
- "I am reading a book that shows me how important it is for me to take a baby aspirin each day. The book also shows me that statins, beta-blockers and ACE inhibitors are not only very effective ways to treat me, but probably even safer than the baby aspirin."
- "Can you tell me any reason why we shouldn't use these medicines to minimize my risk of a heart attack, stroke or even dying young?"

Your doctor may be surprised at the suggestion of an LDL target of under 80. This is not yet widely being discussed, but very recent reports suggest this will become the standard target within the next 5 to 10 years for those with significant risk (which would include smokers). Three recent trials studied people with moderate- to high-dose statin therapy almost without regard to their LDL level at the start of the study (one with simvastatin 40 mg nightly, the Heart Protection Study, and two with atorvastatin 80 mg daily, the AVERT study and MIRACL). Each of these studies demonstrated marked benefit, and the LDL levels achieved by the end of the study were below 80.

Another possibility is that your blood pressure and cholesterol levels are already below these levels. That would be very good news, but would not mean that there is no further cause for concern. Remember that the blood test for cholesterol level is an approximation of what your arteries look like, in terms of their cholesterol content. You need to protect the blood vessels, especially if you still smoke. Low doses of statins and ACE inhibitors can be initiated without dangerous side effects as a vasculoprotective strategy (meaning that they can prevent the development of vascular injury, dysfunction or structural changes). As long as the blood pressure is above 100 (systolic) and the LDL is above 80, the circumstantial evidence supports additional treatment. As an example, the HOPE trial demonstrated marked benefits in midlife adults with vascular disease using a dose of the ACE inhibitor ramipril of 10 mg daily. Perhaps you can take 1.25 or 2.5 mg a day without any side effects, which could help protect your vessels. Similarly, the Heart Protection Study demonstrated that 40 mg nightly of the statin simvastatin markedly reduced risk in those with vascular disease. If your LDL were above 80, 5 or 10 mg nightly is a low dose, associated with extremely low risks, that still has a measurable benefit on cholesterol metabolism.

If you are over the age of 40 with a blood pressure below or near the target of 115/75, you should take aspirin 81 mg daily. Although aspirin is the riskiest of the medicines in this plan, your doctor is likely to recommend it for you. If you have high blood pressure, don't take an aspirin until your pressure gets treated at least down to 140/90, since the risk of bleeding is higher if your blood pressure is very high. If you have high cholesterol, diabetes or a family history of cardiovascular disease, start the aspirin in your 30s. The actual timing should be discussed with your doctor.

Additional targets can provide the extra protection that a smoker needs. As part of the evaluation of your cholesterol, your doctor will also measure the HDL level. This type of cholesterol is good to have at high levels. If your level is low (under 40 for a man and under 50 for a woman), your risks are higher. In contrast, an HDL above these levels significantly reduces your risk. The treatments for low HDL cholesterol have more side effects than the other medicines used in the Before It Happens Plan, and for many people, the side effects of high-dose niacin (yes, the vitamin) are so problematic that it can't be continued. In addition, use of niacin with a statin increases the risk of liver irritation, so close monitoring is needed. Hopefully the ongoing research will lead to a better tolerated and effective treatment for those of you with low HDL levels.

You Still Need to Quit

If you're like most of my patients, you want to quit. You've probably tried to. Your family nags you, you hate the feeling of "needing" a cigarette, and smoking outside at work definitely has major drawbacks. Of the 46 million American adults who smoke, 70 percent—over 30 million—want to quit.

As additional motivation, think of your wallet as well as your health. A typical pack-per-day smoker spends $1,800 to $3,000 each year on cigarettes. With increasing taxes on cigarettes, that number is likely to rise faster than inflation.

"I don't smoke that much anymore," say many of my patients. They seem to think that since they don't smoke "that much," their risk is not so high. Usually this seems to be more of an excuse for not trying to quit rather than something they actually believe.

Fewer than 1 in every 20 people who try to quit smoking are successful.

Because it is so difficult to quit, this plan is particularly suited for you. By implementing this plan, you can cut your risk of heart disease in half even if you continue to smoke. Don't think that means that quitting isn't important. If you continue to smoke, you remain at risk of cancer, and your smoking puts your family at risk, since passive smoking puts them at twice the risk of cardiovascular death.

No one can deal successfully with an addiction or change a long-standing habit unless they are emotionally and intellectually ready. Don't frustrate yourself by trying halfheartedly. You need to be ready to cope with the physical symptoms of nicotine withdrawal as well as the loss of a habit you've had for a number of years. Once you are 100 percent committed, your chance of success is much higher.

The optimist will tell you that quitting is a bit easier than it used to be. In the last decade, the success rate has doubled, although only from 2.5 to 5 percent, as the pessimist will point out. The increased success rate is due in part to a greater acceptance of the link between smoking and disease, which has increased motivation. In addition, there are now some new medicines available that have proven helpful to smokers by lessening the withdrawal effects of quitting.

Though the withdrawal symptoms are relatively mild compared to withdrawal from stronger drugs, the physiological withdrawal process is quite similar. Nicotine withdrawal is not dangerous in the way withdrawal from a drug such as heroin is, but even this minor withdrawal process is a big shock to your body and will be difficult physically and emotionally.

To minimize your discomfort (or torture, depending on your perception of the process), nicotine replacement can be helpful. Some people like wearing a nicotine patch, others prefer the gum since it also provides oral stimulation. After using one of these aids over several weeks or a few months, your body adjusts to life without cigarettes. Both the patch and the gum are available over-the-counter, but you should discuss their use with your doctor. Correct dosage can make the difference between success and failure, so it is important to identify the doses you should use and how quickly to taper off. In both cases, supportive therapy can increase success. But don't think that using a patch or the gum will make this process easy. Using nicotine replacement increases your likelihood of quitting, but it only works when you are committed to quitting.

Some doctors prescribe the medicine bupropion for their patients who are trying to quit. Bupropion was developed as an antidepressant, but it works differently from the more commonly used depression medications (Prozac, Zoloft, Paxil, Celexa etc.) and helps some people quit. As opposed to the nicotine replacements, which a smoker starts using the day he or she quits, bupropion should be started at least two weeks prior to the day you aspire to stop smoking. Because it's a prescription medicine, it's available only through a doctor.

While this medicine is useful, I don't recommend it as strongly as the "core" medicines of this program, aspirin, statins, beta-blockers and ACE inhibitors. Bupropion is not proven to be as safe or well tolerated (worrisome side effects include seizures), and unlike the heart medicines I recommend, it has not been used in millions of people for years and years. However, it's important that you stop smoking, so if you've found no other way to do so, talk to your doctor. He or she can help you evaluate whether or not bupropion is your best option for reaching the important goal of stopping smoking. I would recommend you explore other options for quitting first.

Quitting and Its Affect on Heart Health

Within a year of cessation of smoking, your risk of suffering a heart attack or stroke is cut in half (although still markedly higher than a non-smoker's). In about a decade, your risk becomes the same as that of a non-smoker, assuming you have been lucky enough not to suffer a heart attack within that time period.

Within this plan, you can reduce your risk by at least 50 percent, even if you cannot quit smoking. Quitting provides you additive benefit in reducing your risk of heart attack, stroke and premature death, and together with the medical treatments could reduce your overall risk by nearly 75 percent.

It is difficult to change habits of years and decades. Perhaps one of the approaches currently being studied will eventually make it easy to quit smoking. You know you should quit, but I realize, as you do, that this is a tough task. Therefore, do yourself a favor and give yourself a chance. Adopting this plan now can help ensure that you are still alive at the time when you are ready, willing and able to quit smoking.

The Reality of Smoking

- If you can't quit just yet, then follow this plan to improve your health and reduce your risk of heart disease.
- Your LDL needs to be < 80 using a statin. Your blood pressure needs to be < 115/75.

- Your doctor will choose a statin for your cholesterol, and consider ACE inhibitors, beta-blockers, and possibly a diuretic to keep your blood pressure down.
- Your HgA$_{1c}$ needs to be checked regularly to be sure you show no sign of diabetes.

Once you're emotionally ready to quit, ask your doctor how to proceed.

CHAPTER 13

If You Have HIV

WHEN I WAS IN MEDICAL SCHOOL AND WE PASSED BY ROOMS with HIV patients, we knew we didn't have to worry about their blood pressure or cholesterol levels. They would be dead before there was any chance of developing significant heart disease. In the 20 years since, all that has changed. Today people who are HIV-positive are living longer; long enough to reach midlife and therefore long enough to worry about the usual midlife risks, heart disease being number one among them.

If your viral load is low, your T-cells are okay, and you're tolerating HAART well, your risk of dying of AIDS is much lower than in past years, and in fact, if you're near 50, your risk from AIDS may be lower than your risk from heart disease. Even if you never smoked and have average blood pressure and cholesterol levels, you have lived long enough to reach midlife. This automatically puts you at risk of dying from heart disease. If your cholesterol level or blood pressure is in the range of the typical American adult, then your risk from cardiovascular disease may actually be higher than your risk of dying of AIDS.

From the time you were in your 20s, plaques started to form in the walls of your arteries, and for you—just like for anybody else—the likelihood of the plaques causing a problem increases with age. While some studies suggest that your plaques may get worse from the HIV infection or your antiretroviral therapy (especially protease inhibitors), these effects are small compared to the risks that come with reaching

> When it comes to heart disease, you're just like anybody else—at high risk by the time you reach middle age.

the age of 50. (See below for more information about a possible relationship between HIV, your medicines, and heart disease.) The key factor is that you have led a typical adult life, with new plaques forming and old plaques growing silently since your 20s.

You may be unaware that you have heart disease, but if you are near 50, you probably do. Whether you have heart disease, high blood pressure or high cholesterol, you don't need to change your anti-HIV regimen—it's working and you should continue to benefit from what it does for you. This plan can be implemented alongside your anti-HIV regimen and provide marked reduction in your risk of a heart attack or premature death by up to 50 percent or more.

The Plan for People with HIV

• LDL cholesterol under 100, if possible.
• Blood pressure less than 115/75.
• If your heart has hypertrophy or weakness based on an ECG or echocardiogram, you need a beta-blocker.
• If you have additional risk factors, you need an ACE inhibitor to protect your blood vessels.
• If you are diabetic, a glycohemoglobin of under 6%.

Heart Disease and the HIV Patient

HIV infection and antiretroviral treatments appear to increase the risk of cardiovascular disease, but do so only slightly. The amount of risk is small compared to the benefit of antiretroviral therapy and can be minimized with this plan.

In the late 1980s, investigators observed that HIV infection was associated with abnormalities of cholesterol metabolism that could increase cardiovascular risk (elevations in the level of triglycerides, a type of cholesterol that increases risk, but much less so than increases in LDL cholesterol).

In the early 1990s, data suggested a link between anti-HIV medications and the development of cardiovascular disease. Soon after, several other reports emerged describing specific molecular mechanisms whereby HIV infection could contribute further to the development of cardiovascular disease. HIV can kill the endothelial cells that line the blood vessel walls, which are crucial to maintaining stability of the cover overlying the cholesterol-filled plaques. Any change in the biologic or structural integrity of this cap on the plaque makes rupture more likely (this is what causes a heart attack or sudden death).

In order to quantify the potential effect of the infection and the medications on cardiovascular risk, a group of investigators recently published an analysis of the clinical course of over 35,000 people treated for HIV infection within the last decade. The study included people who received nucleoside analogs, protease inhibitors, and nonnucleoside reverse-transcriptase inhibitors, with many receiving combinations of these therapies (in recent years HAART).

The study demonstrated that none of the medications, alone or in combination, significantly increased the risk of cardiovascular disease. There was no relationship between the duration of antiretroviral therapy and cardiovascular risks, which was a reassuring sign that continued HIV treatment does not significantly alter the risk-benefit ratio. The highest risk was in people who had preexisting cholesterol or blood pressure problems, as well as those with diabetes or a history of smoking.

Are you a candidate for the Before It Happens Plan?
•••

Vicki is 58 and has been HIV-positive for 8 years. She has smoked for years, and it would seem that her blood pressure seems good (135/80). At her age, with her smoking history and her blood pressure, her HIV infection has little to do with her risk of cardiovascular problems. When Vicki starts on an aspirin, statin, beta-blocker and ACE inhibitor, her risk will be reduced by 75 percent.

Therefore, people who are HIV-infected should continue to treat themselves aggressively against the virus. The downside is that as HIV treatment increases in effectiveness, HIV patients are more prone to live long enough to develop more advanced and life-threatening cardiovascular disease, just because of the changes that occur in our blood vessels by the time we reach midlife.

It is no longer a question of whether people who are HIV-positive develop cardiovascular disease, but rather of how they can be treated to prevent heart attacks or strokes. The Before It Happens Plan can be individualized for you, accounting for your HIV and the medicines you must take.

The Plan for People with HIV

You're already living with one challenging illness, and I'm sorry to have to tell you that you also have to worry about cardiovascular disease, too. However, if you look at the bright side of things, it's terrific that people with HIV are making it to midlife and have to be concerned about the same things everyone else does.

If you are a 50-year-old man with total cholesterol of 221, LDL cholesterol of 143 and blood pressure of 135/80, your risk of a myocardial infarction or cardiovascular death in the next 10 years is 8 percent; almost a 1 in 100 chance of having a heart attack during the next year. 1 of 4 men dies within a year of his first heart attack, so that means you have a 1 in 500 chance of dying in less than 2 years from a heart attack. That should not seem like a low risk to you.

If you were a 50-year-old woman with the same cholesterol and blood pressure, your risk of a heart attack in the next 10 years would be 2 percent. Within a year of a heart attack, 38 percent of women die, giving you a 1 in 1,300 chance of dying from a heart attack in less than 2 years. While this is lower than for men, this risk is still about 4 to 5 times higher than risk of dying in a car accident. You wouldn't drive without seatbelts, would you?

In both cases, the risks can be brought down considerably. Lowering the blood pressure or cholesterol to optimal levels would each reduce that risk by 50 percent, and lowering both successfully would reduce the risk by 75 percent.

As you know from reading other parts of the book, I don't want you to be satisfied with "average" healthcare. Anyone who has battled their way through HIV deserves to be treated optimally for heart disease. If there are safe and easy ways to reduce these risks by 50 to 75 percent, don't you want to know about them? In Chapter 4, I reviewed the scientific evidence showing how safe and effective the medicines in the plan are, and in Part 2 advised you how to work with your doctor as a partner.

The Before It Happens Plan for those with HIV still includes each of the four main pharmacological components: low-dose aspirin, a statin, a beta-blocker and an ACE inhibitor. However, in contrast to the other people on the Before It Happens program, the selection of drugs and their doses needs to be considered carefully owing to the increased possibility of drug interactions and adverse effects.

Insist on Optimal Protection

Be specific about your expectations, and realize that because of the medicines you are taking, you should limit yourself to the specific medicines listed.

Your doctor may be surprised at the suggestion of an LDL target of under 100 if you don't have diabetes or haven't already suffered a heart attack. Studies show that your risk is lower if your LDL is lower, and statins reduce LDL safely. Even if your LDL doesn't change much, if you have no side effects from your statin, you should continue it because it can still have beneficial effects on the plaques in your blood vessels, and that will reduce your risk.

Ideally, you should be treated with additional medications if your HDL were low or your triglycerides high. Since the medicines used for these two problems are metabolized in your liver and not as safe or simple to use as statins, you should discuss with your doctor how to individualize your plan, which may include the need to visit a specialist in cholesterol management.

Blood pressure control is just as important; your blood pressure should be 115/75. As with the statins, you cannot take any one of the medicines of a given type; instead, selection will be based on the potential for drug interactions and liver metabolism. Reducing blood pressure by 20 points will cut your risk of heart attacks and strokes in half. It's worth the effort.

Although the battle against HIV is far from over, the successes are so remarkable that you need to consider other health risks. That means that once you near midlife (50), you need to adopt a strategy of preventive medical care that should focus primarily on your risk of heart disease. Implementing the Before It Happens Plan will reduce your risk substantially, providing a longer and healthier future.

Insist on Optimal Protection for Yourself

- Statins reduce the fat deposits in your plaques, reduce the likelihood of rupture and improve vessel function.
- ACE inhibitors improve vascular function and enhance plaque stability.
- Beta-blockers prevent heart arrhythmias and reduce the risk of sudden death in people with coronary artery disease (especially those with a history of a heart attack), high blood pressure or heart failure.

- "I am reading a book that explains that my risk of a heart attack or stroke is likely to be higher than my risk of dying from HIV. Can you estimate the percent chance that I will become disabled or die from an HIV-related illness in the next two years?"
- "According to the Framingham study, as a 50-year-old man with the typical blood pressure and cholesterol levels of an average American, I have almost a 1 percent chance of having a heart attack in the next year, and a 25 percent chance of dying within the year following a heart attack." (If you go to the website of the

NIH, at http://hin.nhlbi.nih.gov/atpiii/calculator.asp?user-type=prof, you can calculate your risk—although it reports your 10-year risk, just divide by 10 for your annual risk.)

- "Since lowering my blood pressure and my LDL cholesterol would reduce those risks, would I be a candidate for these medicines?

  1. Aspirin, 81 mg daily,

  2. The statin pravastatin,

  3. The beta-blocker atenolol [or carvedilol if you have diabetes that is not well controlled], and

  4. The ACE inhibitor ramipril or lisinopril"

The Importance of the Right Combination of Medicines with HIV Infection
••••••••••••••••••••••••••••••••••

For anyone who is being treated for HIV, a prescribing doctor needs to carefully consider the patient's mix of medicines. Antiretroviral therapies can interact directly with many medicines in a fashion that can reduce their effectiveness or increase their risks. (You are all too familiar with the need to adjust dosages and change from one medicine to another, both within a class and between different classes.)

Since most antiretroviral therapies are metabolized in the liver, your doctor must consider the effects of prescribing drugs that are metabolized by the same enzymes because of the possibility of a negative interaction. (If you also have a history of hepatitis, you need to pay careful attention to what medicines you are taking.) The key point in liver metabolism of antiretroviral medications is the cytochrome P450 3A4 enzyme (referred to as 3A4). If your doctor can avoid any medicines that rely on the 3A4 system, this will reduce the risk of drug interactions and side effects.

The information that follows details why certain drugs may be preferred over others in the same class.

Statin:

Although any statin can be used to treat cholesterol, the HIV patient receiving antiretroviral therapy, will fare best with pravastatin. This is the statin with the largest safety record that is not metabolized in a 3A4 system (in contrast with the other statins). Although pravastatin is not as potent as some of the other statins, and you and your doctor could be disappointed by the relatively small changes in blood levels of cholesterol, remember that this is not the whole story. The key target is not the blood level but rather the lipid in the arterial wall. Even if your blood tests are not markedly better, pravastatin (especially at higher doses) markedly decreases your risk of a heart attack or stroke. Using pravastatin is a safe choice because it has little risk of drug interactions or irritation of your liver.

Beta-Blocker:

If you have diabetes or insulin resistance, the optimal beta-blocker for you is carvedilol. It is primarily metabolized in the liver through the cytochrome P450 2D6 system, but there is some metabolism through the 3A4 system. The reason that this is the first choice for those of you with diabetes (or pre-diabetes) is its benefit on glucose metabolism and insulin sensitivity. In contrast to other beta-blockers, carvedilol slightly but significantly improves diabetes control compared to two other beta-blockers. This benefit outweighs the small potential risk for drug interactions. In addition, carvedilol reduced the risk of death compared to metoprolol in patients with heart failure in the only trial in cardiovascular medicine to directly compare two medicines in the same class. Clearly, carvedilol is a superior beta-blocker.

(continued on page 176)

(continued from page 175)

Because protease inhibitors for your HIV could make you more sensitive to the effect of a beta-blocker, you will require a smaller beta-blocker dose to start with and likely would not require such a high dose long-term. If you have any history suggesting impairment or dysfunction of your liver, your beta-blocker choice should be atenolol, since it is not metabolized through the liver. In general, without diabetes, atenolol should be your first choice.

ACE Inhibitor:

For most patients, ACE inhibitors do not appear to be metabolized significantly by the 3A4 system, making the selection of which one to use less critical. However, I would advocate using "once daily" drugs, preferably those that have a property called tissue avidity. Although ramipril (used in the HOPE trial) seems like a good choice, it is metabolized in your liver. With the potential for liver irritation with your HIV medications, it may be best to avoid any more drugs that could affect your liver.

Certainly, if you also have significant liver dysfunction, as can be the case if you have chronic hepatitis or a history of hepatitis in the past, your ACE inhibitor should be lisinopril instead. This is also a drug that requires only once-daily administration and has a large and convincing safety record. Ramipril has the theoretical advantage of being tissue avid, which may improve vascular health. Lisinopril does not have this property, but still is proven safe and effective and, importantly, is not metabolized in the liver.

The Reality of HIV

- Just like anyone else, you are at risk of heart disease by the time you reach middle age.
- Your LDL needs to be < 100. Your blood pressure needs to be < 115/75.

- Because of the medicines you are already on for HIV, your doctor needs to make a very careful selection of medications. Your doctor will choose a statin for your cholesterol and consider ACE inhibitors (preferably lisinopril), beta-blockers (preferably atenolol), and possibly a diuretic to keep your blood pressure down.
- With your doctor's okay, you should be taking an aspirin (81 mg) a day.
- Your HgA_{1c} needs to be checked regularly to be certain you aren't showing signs of diabetes.

CHAPTER 14

Men: You Are At Risk

OF THE 1,100,000 PEOPLE WHO SUFFER A HEART ATTACK EACH year, 250,000 people will not even have time to call 9-1-1 before dying suddenly. Most of them are men.

If you're like most men hitting midlife, then you've slowly begun to think about heart disease. Most men don't like to admit that they're worried, but when they are in my office and we start to talk about their health, they'll tell me a personal story that caught their attention—something that happened to a friend or a neighbor. Maybe that's what got you thinking, too. Perhaps you became worried when you overheard your colleague speaking of his cousin who dropped dead unexpectedly. Or maybe you had a friend like mine, a fit man in his early 50s, who died suddenly soon after returning from his daily jog.

Your concerns are well based. Just ask the family of Jim Fixx, the marathon runner who made jogging an American pastime before dropping dead from a heart attack at age 52. Or perhaps you heard about the major league pitcher Darryl Kile, dead from heart disease at 33. No one is immune—not even heart experts. Jeff Isner, a leading scientist in the field of gene therapy for heart disease, suffered a fatal heart attack at 52.

Heart disease affects the young and middle-aged, not just the elderly. The average age of a man having his first heart attack is only 66. Almost half of those who suffer their first heart attack under the age of 65 will be dead within eight years. That means if you suffer a heart attack at the age of 60, you only have a 50 percent chance of making it to 68. According to U.S. government data, a typical 60-year-old who

The Plan for Men
••••••••••••••••••••

- Your LDL needs to be < 100.
- Your blood pressure needs to be < 115/75 (both numbers).
- You need an ACE inhibitor to protect your blood vessels (vascular health).
- You need a beta-blocker if your ECG or echocardiogram suggests hypertrophy or weakness of your heart.
- You need to take an aspirin (81 mg) each day.
- You need your HDL > 40.
- If you have diabetes, you need your HgA_{1c} to be < 6%.

does not suffer a heart attack has a 50 percent chance of making it to age 85. That's seventeen years' difference in life expectancy.

If you are 50 (or getting close) or your blood pressure and cholesterol levels are not perfect, then you are at a higher risk than you need to be. Implementing this plan will reduce your risk of heart attack, stroke and premature death. The plan is easy, with no diets and no stress about trying to get out of work in time to get to the gym. Based on your condition, you can start to cut your risk now. The four medicines in this program are proven safe and will reduce your risk. In fact, these medicines are safer than standard vitamins.

Are you a candidate for the Before It Happens Plan?
••

Bob is 56 and at the top of his career. He exercises regularly. But he also has a high LDL—not that high, but high enough. He also has the typical blood pressure for a man in his 50s, 128/85. He already takes a baby aspirin a day to prevent a heart attack. By adding a statin and an ACE inhibitor, his risk is cut in half.

50-Year-Old Blood Vessels

By the time you reach 50, you have a lot of plaques in your coronary arteries. You can't tell, but several studies prove that they are there (and have been since you were in your 20s). Doctors at the Cleveland Clinic inserted a special catheter into the arteries of the hearts in over 300 people, and through this catheter passed a wire with a small ultrasound machine on the tip. They found that nearly three quarters of people over 40 and 85 percent of those over 50 had significant plaques in their coronary arteries; and these were people who were thought to have perfect hearts.

These plaques weren't filled with calcium, which would be detectable with the new CAT scanners. Calcium is deposited late in the development of coronary artery disease, so a positive calcium score on an ultrafast CAT scan or electron beam CAT scan is bad news, but a score of zero is not necessarily good news. In fact, a man in his 50s (and most in their 40s) will have coronary artery disease even with a score of zero.

Another way to diagnose coronary artery disease is for you to have a stress test, usually performed by taking pictures of your heart before and after exercise. This is useful for finding evidence of big plaques in your coronary arteries, ones that block most blood flow. These big plaques cause symptoms, but usually do not cause heart attacks.

The dangerous plaques are the small ones, and you have a lot of these throughout the arteries in your heart. Because almost everyone over 50 has these plaques and the treatments are so safe, everyone should be treated to stabilize these plaques and prevent ruptures.

Fifty-year-old blood vessels undergo another change, one that should be easy to visualize. They aren't as flexible as they used to be, just like the rest of you. Along with this change comes a gradual increase in blood pressure, with the average man having a blood pressure that is not considered high blood pressure by the standard definition, but is too high to be considered normal by anyone (the average systolic blood pressure for an American man in his 50s is 125). This adds to your risk of a plaque rupture.

Most doctors don't think much about a blood pressure of 125/85, but when your pressure starts to rise, your future is predictable—you will develop high blood pressure. You need to start treatment early, as soon as your blood pressure is no longer optimal (above 115/75) in order to minimize your risk and help the blood vessels return to their normal flexible and compliant state.

If your blood pressure is a little high, your cholesterol is not perfect, you weigh 10 to 15 percent more than your ideal body weight or someone in your family has heart disease, then the odds of having plaques go even higher. The study from the Cleveland Clinic showed the same thing as studies from trauma victims and war casualties, your plaques are small, cholesterol-filled bumps, frequently with evidence of inflammation. To stabilize them and prevent rupture, you need to implement the Before It Happens Plan.

How High Is Your Risk?

What if your risk of a heart attack, stroke, or death in the next year were about 1 percent? Does that seem like a high risk to you? If you are a 56-year-old man with optimal blood pressure (115/75) and decent cholesterol levels (total cholesterol of 195, HDL of 43 and LDL of 117), your risk of a heart attack in the next year is 0.8 percent, and you have a 25 percent chance of dying within a year of that heart attack.

That means you have a 1 in 500 chance of dying from a heart attack in the next two years. Compare this risk to your lifetime chance of dying in a car crash (1 in 6,585), a plane crash (1 in 659,779) or a residential fire (1 in 83,025). You wear seatbelts, are reassured by airbags and have smoke detectors installed (go check your batteries if you can't remember the last time you did). Don't you think you should pay as much attention to preventing a heart attack?

According to standard guidelines, an acceptable cholesterol level is associated with a 25 percent to 35 percent higher risk than an optimal level. Acceptable blood pressure is associated with two to three times as many heart attacks, strokes and deaths compared to optimal blood pressure.

It's not that no one wants to protect you. In fact, midlife men should take specific steps to prevent a heart attack. The standard guidelines from both medical societies and federal government panels tell your doctor to prescribe a baby aspirin (81 mg) for you to take every day to prevent heart attacks, even if you are given a clean bill of health. Studies prove that aspirin is safe, especially for men around age 50 or older, when the risk of a heart attack starts to rise significantly. Aspirin therapy reduces your risk of a heart attack by about 25 percent.

At the risk of being redundant, this recommendation from the standard guidelines is great, but stops short of minimizing the danger you face as a middle-aged man. Instead of limiting your treatment to strategies that are affordable to society, this plan focuses on those treatments that are safe and effective for you.

Once you refuse to be treated only at an "acceptable" level and commit to optimal care with optimal control of your blood pressure, cholesterol and vascular health, you are well on your way to staying alive and healthy.

Implementing The Plan

If your doctor tells you that your blood pressure or cholesterol levels are abnormal, or even if they are borderline, your next step is straightforward. Tell your doctor you don't want your levels high, you don't even want them on the borderline, you want them optimal, and then your risk will be minimized. When discussing the following issues with your doctor, select the parts of the text within the brackets that relate to you.

- "I understand that having high levels of [cholesterol and/or blood pressure], or even borderline levels, means my risk of a heart attack or stroke is higher than it could be."
- "Since medicines such as [statins, beta-blockers, ACE inhibitors] are so safe, and can help me have optimal [cholesterol and/or blood pressure], can I start taking them now?"

- "I know you may need to take more blood tests and have me visit more often, but I am willing because I understand my risk is minimized when my LDL cholesterol is under 100 and my blood pressure under 115/75."
- "Since I am over 50, should I follow the standard recommendation to take a baby aspirin each day to prevent a heart attack?"

There is nothing magical about starting the plan when you reach 50. I chose 50 because that is what most studies choose. But some choose 45 and show the same thing—that your risk starts to climb between 40 and 50 years of age, even without any evidence of abnormal blood pressure or cholesterol levels. If you feel more comfortable being more aggressive, start sooner.

Mike is 42, but he wanted to get control of his health right away. His doctor told him he was fine. He didn't smoke or have diabetes, and no one in his family has heart disease. But Mike's blood pressure was 130/80 and his LDL was 131. According to the standard guidelines, Mike should modify his lifestyle, and that's all. But he works long hours, and just can't seem to get to the gym or find the time to prepare the healthiest meals. Since starting on low doses of a statin, a beta-blocker and an ACE inhibitor, in addition to taking a baby aspirin, his risk is almost 70 percent lower.

If you have a relative who has heart disease, you are overweight (even 10 to 15 percent) or smoke, you should start this plan earlier. In those cases, look at the chapter that's relevant to you for further information.

The Hard Part of The Plan

When he turned 50, Douglas decided it was time to get his heart evaluated again. A few years before, he had what is referred to as a comprehensive executive physical. He had blood tests, an electrocardiogram and a stress test. He was quite proud of his performance on the stress test, which showed that his consistent exercise was keeping him in good physical condition. However, Douglas had a problem; he smoked a pack of cigarettes a day for years.

I explained to Douglas that the normal stress test was reassuring, but that it couldn't detect the kind of problems in his heart that would be most likely for a smoker, and the most dangerous. Douglas probably had many fatty, inflamed plaques in his arteries. These are the plaques that don't cause symptoms and aren't detectable by a stress test; they are also the ones that are most likely to rupture and cause a heart attack or sudden death. His blood pressure was 110/70, but his cholesterol profile included an LDL of 117. Douglas needed a statin to minimize his risk, but it wouldn't be enough.

Even though his blood pressure was optimal, all those cigarettes had damaged the cells lining his arteries, making his plaques even more likely to rupture. An ACE inhibitor would help stabilize those plaques and restore normal function to his blood vessels. Even though his blood pressure was low, Douglas's vascular system needed protection, and an ACE inhibitor would help.

I explained to Douglas what had happened and would continue to happen to his arteries, and advised him to start an aspirin, a statin and an ACE inhibitor, and, of course, to stop smoking cigarettes. His risk of a heart attack was 1.2 percent in the next year a 1 in 83 chance of a heart attack within the year. If he quits, his odds improve to 1 in 166 (risk cut in half). If he takes the aspirin, statin and ACE inhibitor, the risk drops to 1 in 250 even if he doesn't quit smoking, or 1 in 500 if he takes the medicines and quits. Douglas understood the math, he knew that he had two options; he could do either or both, and as long as he did anything, he would be much better off.

Intellectually, Douglas understood what he needed to do, but he couldn't do either. He said he was worried about gaining weight if he quit. He said he was scared of taking medicines, because that was what "old people" did. He knew how simple his choices were, but he seemed afraid to make the commitment.

Each time I see Douglas, we have the same discussion. He has many reasons why he can't take that simple first step. We discuss different strategies for quitting cigarettes, different reasons why he needs to start on these medicines, especially since he is not ready to quit smoking. All the while, he continues to exercise, but also continues in a highly stressful and all-consuming job. Despite his attempts to watch his diet, his LDL is now 124.

I hope Douglas will be ready to take control of his health soon. I plan to give him a copy of this book, but I think his wife is more likely to read it than he is. I just hope I can convince Douglas to do something before his heart attack. Once he has a heart attack, he really increases his risk of dying young, with a 50 percent chance of being dead within 8 years. Hopefully, you are more ready than Douglas to start this plan.

Lifestyle Changes Are Secondary

Many of my colleagues enjoy telling me that lifestyle changes are the most important steps to take. I agree with the importance, but I don't believe it is necessarily the first intervention. Lifestyle changes provide relatively minor benefits compared to those of the medical therapies of this plan. Perhaps more important, people cannot make major lifestyle changes with consistency (pardon the generalization if you are one of the few who can).

Few people have time to exercise regularly; they are busy getting the kids to school or racing home for dinner to see the family before collapsing for the night. In Chapter 17 I will suggest some simple ways to increase your exercise. Why not walk to work? Why not use the parking lot a bit further away, or use the stairs instead of the elevator? If people kept their diets the same, and exercised enough to burn off 10 or 15 extra calories a day, the typical increase in weight in our 40s and 50s could be prevented. It doesn't take much.

Plain and simple, it is tough to change habits. Don't use all your energy fighting this reality. Start with the easy things you can do to reduce your risk and then gradually figure out how to work on the harder parts. The Before It Happens Plan provides you with the way to reduce risks starting now, simply and safely. Make the commitment and get started.

Men: The Reality of Your Risk

- Heart disease affects the young and middle-aged, not just the elderly. You need to talk about your personal risk factors with your doctor now.

- If you're over 50, or near 50, your cholesterol and blood pressure numbers need to be optimal: LDL < 100; blood pressure < 115/75; HDL > 40.

- Your doctor will choose a statin for your cholesterol and consider ACE inhibitors, beta-blockers and possibly a diuretic to keep your blood pressure down.

- Lifestyle changes are secondary, but they are still important to consider as you age.

CHAPTER 15

Women Are At Risk Too

WHAT DO YOU WORRY ABOUT? IF YOU'RE LIKE MOST WOMEN I know, you worry about the people around you—your kids, your husband and your parents. Your friends' needs sometimes seem more important than your own. You probably read the chapters in this book that apply to everyone else before you turned to this one. I'm glad you're concerned about your family and friends, but right now I want you to be selfish and think about yourself.

But I bet I still don't have your full attention. Unfortunately, when it comes to worrisome health issues, my subject—the heart—is not the first one women think of. Instead, worries of breast cancer predominate. As a man, I cannot feel the emotional impact of worrying about breast cancer. I do know the illness is devastating physically and emotionally—and the risk is high. That's why your doctor recommends regular mammograms, which enable detection of disease earlier, when it is easier to treat and when the treatment you require is easier on you.

You Need to Pay Attention Now

It's going to be tough to get your attention: but you need to know. You are more likely to get heart disease than cancer, and more likely to become disabled or die from cardiovascular disease than cancer. Just ask actress Sharon Stone; not even 50, she was stricken by a stroke. Good luck and the fact that she got to a hospital quickly were all that kept her from dying—and she had never been diagnosed with cardiovascular disease.

These doctors are lucky. The public is so well informed on the subject of screening for breast cancer that the only controversy generally involves when to start baseline mammograms and whether to have them yearly or every other year. I want you to be informed about your heart also. Here's why.

Heart Disease: Bigger Risk than Breast Cancer

When you stack up the statistics for breast cancer and for heart disease, it is rather sobering to realize that heart disease is a bigger problem to women over the age of 40—and certainly over the age of 50—than breast cancer. As reported by the organization WomenHeart, 1 out of every 10 women between the ages of 45 and 64—over 3.1 million—suffer from one form or another of heart disease. Each year 194,000 women are diagnosed with breast cancer and 41,000 die annually, while more than double that—435,000 women—suffer heart attacks each year; and 83,000 of those are under the age of 65. A shocking 9,000 women who have heart attacks are under the age of 45.

Still not convinced? Consider Figure 15.1, which compares the number of women affected by invasive breast cancer and those diagnosed with coronary artery disease. According to the National Cancer Institute, for women in their 40s the likelihood of having breast cancer is 0.75 percent, or 75 of every 10,000, and for those in their 50s it is 1.83 percent, or 183 of every 10,000. The American Heart Association reports that 2.8 percent of women between 25 and 44 years of age have coronary disease, as do 5.5 percent between 45 and 54. That means that 280 of every 10,000 women 25 to 44 years of age and 550 of every 10,000 women between 45 and 54 years of age have coronary disease. That's seven times more women with heart disease in their 40s and 50s than are diagnosed with breast cancer. As you can see, these statistics merit your attention.

If there is good news in any of this, it is that the treatments for heart disease are effective and well tolerated. The medicines in this plan reduce the risk of sudden death as well as the risk of chronic heart dis-

Women Have Coronary Disease
Much More Commonly than Breast Cancer

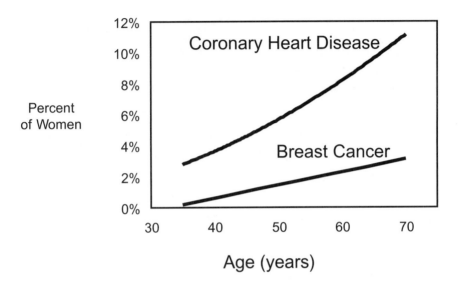

Figure 15.1 Most women think they're safe if they escape breast cancer. Did you know that more than 20 times more women get coronary artery disease, even in their 40s and 50s?

ease, or, as my patients say, they will make you live longer. Few women think twice about taking vitamins. The medicines in this program are safer than many vitamins.

Women Are Treated Differently from Men

The American Heart Association points out that, despite the fact that more women die of heart disease than men, women are less likely to receive optimal treatments after a heart attack. Statistics show that women get only a third as many stents placed, only a quarter as many defibrillators implanted, and just over a third as many open-heart operations as men. In essence, women are not treated as aggressively when it comes to either the selection of diagnostic tests or treatments.

The Plan for Women

....

- Your LDL needs to be < 100.
- Your blood pressure needs to be < 115/75 (both numbers).
- You need an ACE inhibitor to protect your blood vessels once you reach menopause.
- You need to take an aspirin (81 mg) each day once you reach menopause.
- You need your HDL > 50.
- If you have diabetes, you need your HgA_{1c} to be < 6%.

- The two medicines that are first choices are ACE inhibitors and beta-blockers, because each reduces your risk more than just by lowering blood pressure (ARB may be substituted for ACE inhibitors if you can't tolerate them). The next choice should be a diuretic.

Critics might blame the predominantly male medical profession for gender bias in treatment, however, I don't think that doctors set out to deal with women differently. If you look closely at the data, it becomes clear that the differences are due largely to the fact that heart disease presents differently in women. If there is blame to be laid, it might well have to do with the fact that more studies have been conducted on men than on women, so that we better understand how cardiovascular disease evolves and causes symptoms in men. Women present with symptoms that are less likely to be recognized for the warning signs that they are. You need to take charge and make sure that your doctor understands you and your symptoms.

This book is your call to action. If you understand your own gender-specific warning signs, you will be better prepared to advocate for yourself.

Plaque Problem: Different in Women

Heart attacks are caused by two distinct mechanisms, both of which lead to reduced blood flow to the heart muscle. Part of the reason that the symptoms of heart disease may be different than for men is that women can suffer heart attacks caused by a different mechanism.

The first and most commonly described cause of a heart attack (and the one that occurs primarily in males) happens as a result of a break in the thin lining that covers a fatty plaque (made up of cholesterol) in the artery wall. Initially, a small break may heal and not be noticed externally, but it may cause a slight disturbance in the blood flow, much as a large rock in a stream might slightly divert the water flow while still letting the water get by. However, some plaques may be inflamed and filled with cholesterol. When these plaques rupture, the material within the plaque causes a dense blood clot, which can completely block the blood flow in the artery, like a large boulder in a small stream blocking the flow totally. A complete and abrupt obstruction in your coronary arteries will lead to a heart attack and potentially an arrhythmia that could be instantly fatal.

If the first plaque rupture is not fatal, then more and more small ruptures may occur, leading to severe blockages. Eventually blood flow will be affected and symptoms will develop. At this advanced stage, any stress test will detect these severe blockages.

Are you a candidate for the Before It Happens Plan?

Ana is 48. She stays in shape, is not overweight and doesn't smoke. Her blood pressure is ideal, but her cholesterol level isn't quite optimal. Ana's risk is high because she is about to enter menopause and because of her family history. Ana's dad died from a heart attack at 42. Taking an aspirin and a statin will cut her risk almost in half.

In women, the most common cause of a heart attack is an erosion on the thin lining covering the plaques. The erosion can be quite small, but an inflamed cholesterol-filled plaque can activate the immune and blood-clotting systems quickly, leading to blood clot formation and alteration of blood flow within the artery. The clinical effects can be more subtle than those that occur when a plaque ruptures, and this is considered a major reason why women's symptoms present differently.

Heart Attack Symptoms Present Differently in Women

Newspapers and television programs frequently do helpful features about warning signs of heart attack. Yet almost all of these stories present only the male point of view, that the standard presenting symptom is chest pain. The medical term for this symptom is *angina pectoris,* a Latin phrase that means chest discomfort. Although many patients report the symptom as painful, others describe it as pressure or heaviness. The pain may radiate from the left side of the chest to the left arm or even up into the neck or the jaw.

For women, chest pain or chest pressure is not always the predominant symptom of a heart attack. A woman's first sign may be shortness of breath, nausea, neck or jaw pain or fatigue. A change in your ability to exercise is also a major warning sign for women, as I explain later in this chapter. At times, a woman may also describe a slight amount of chest discomfort.

At the risk of making a generalization that I cannot support with scientific evidence, I believe that women do not react to pain the way men do: they do experience discomfort but are less likely to complain about it. A colleague once told me that this is obviously true. After all, he pointed out, do you think that any family would have more than one child if men were the ones to carry and deliver? When it comes to a heart attack, however, speaking up is a good thing. Usually a woman having a heart attack who at first does not describe chest pain may later admit that perhaps there was a slight bit of discomfort.

Pay Attention to a Change in Exercise Capacity

If you exercise regularly you are at a lower risk of heart attack and stroke. You also provide yourself with a way to gauge whether you may be developing cardiovascular disease. Even subtle changes in cardiovascular function can make you consciously or unconsciously exercise less vigorously. You may tell yourself that you've been stressed at work or that the cold weather has kept you indoors and you think you're just out of shape—check in with your doctor anyway. While the doctor may be able to reassure you that it's something else, you don't want to find out later that coronary artery disease was the cause.

In Chapter 1 I told you about the 39-year-old woman who noticed difficulty keeping up with her children. She also had borderline blood pressure, and was advised to alter her lifestyle, as recommended by the standard guidelines. Unfortunately, she suffered a significant heart attack a few weeks later, and I met her as she was undergoing an emergency angioplasty. It was fortunate that she came to the emergency room right away. It was less than three hours from the onset of her first symptoms until her vessel was opened. Nonetheless, she had sustained a significant heart attack—and had a 38 percent chance of dying within a year and a 50 percent chance within 8 years.

Despite her youth, I would have treated this woman with the medicines in this plan, based on her borderline blood pressure and her reduced exercise capacity. But I wonder whether she might also have been treated differently if she were a he. It is more common for men than for women to receive medications and to undergo catheter-based procedures and operations when presenting to doctors with either typical or atypical symptoms.

Feeling tired or having a reduced capacity for exercise is a somewhat surprising, but very real, symptom of a heart attack in women. Most doctors act as though this is a problem that can be ignored. If you experience these symptoms, you cannot afford to ignore them. The symptoms women experience with cardiovascular disease may be different from those of men, and both you and your doctor need to understand these differences. Talk about it at your next appointment.

- "I understand from this book I am reading that men and women have different symptoms of heart disease."
- "Can you explain how I should react to these different symptoms?"
- "How do you change your approach when treating women?"

You would understand your doctor's responsiveness to less typical symptoms if you ask about one now. For example:

- "I know it may have nothing to do with my heart, but I have been aware of feeling fatigued over the past few months (or whatever time period applies to you). Since fatigue can be a presenting symptom of a weak heart, can you send me in for an echocardiogram to learn with certainty whether I have heart disease?"

Plan Basics

You must insist on getting treatment that is as good as—if not better than—what a man would get.

If your doctor tells you that your blood pressure or cholesterol levels are abnormal, or even if they are borderline, your next step is pretty straightforward. Tell your doctor you don't want your levels high, you don't even want them on the borderline, you want them optimal, and then your risk will be minimized. When discussing the following issues with your doctor, select the parts of the text within the brackets that relate to you.

- "I understand that having high levels of [cholesterol and/or blood pressure], or even borderline levels, means my risk of a heart attack or stroke is higher than it could be."
- "Since medicines such as [statins, beta-blockers, ACE inhibitors] are so safe, and can help me have optimal [cholesterol and/or blood pressure], can I start taking them now?"

- "I know you may need to take more blood tests and have me visit more often, but I am willing because I understand my risk is minimized when my LDL cholesterol is under 100 and my blood pressure under 115/75."

- "Since I am over 50, should I follow the standard recommendation to take a baby aspirin each day to prevent a heart attack, and if not, why not?"

There is nothing magical about starting the plan when you reach 50. I chose 50 because it is a time when most of us take stock of our lives. If you have a relative who has heart disease, are overweight (even 10 to 15 percent), smoke or have begun the process of menopause, you should start this plan. In those cases, look at the chapter that's relevant to you for further information.

Even if all your numbers are optimal, you should talk to your doctor about starting low-dose aspirin therapy (81 mg a day has the same benefits as but less risk than 325 mg a day). Despite the fact that aspirin is an over-the-counter drug, its use should be discussed with your doctor (as should all of the medications in the plan).

The medicines that form the basis for the plan are extremely well tolerated and very safe. You should expect to experience minimal, if any, side effects, although this may require adjustment of doses and perhaps even selection of different medicines within the same family of related medicines.

Hormone Replacement Therapy (HRT)

Up until recently, many premenopausal women have been treated with hormone replacement therapy to reduce the symptoms of menopause. While HRT was prescribed to help women stave off symptoms of menopause, it soon became promoted as a way to prevent cardiovascular disease, which unfortunately did not prove to be true. Only within the past few years have any studies actually tested the safety of hormone replacement. Two randomized, placebo-controlled trials indicated that hormone replacement was potentially dangerous. One study (Women's Health Initiative) showed an increase in heart attacks, strokes, blood clots and breast cancer, while the other (Heart and Estrogen-Progestin Replacement Study) reported that women with established heart disease were at an increased risk of heart attacks during the first year of use, although over time, the amount of risk decreased in magnitude. Even the major health benefits—reduced risk of osteoporosis and improved cholesterol balance—can be achieved more effectively and safely by other medicines. Therefore, the only reason to consider the use of hormone replacement therapy is for treatment of debilitating symptoms from menopause, short-term, for a woman willing to accept all the risks.

Many postmenopausal women are already taking hormone replacement therapy because they started it before these two recent studies were completed. Stopping hormone replacement therapy has been difficult for many of the patients in my practice, because most are convinced (as many doctors have been) that this is a safe, effective and important therapy. I saw a patient recently, Lori, who is 68 and suffers from high blood pressure. For the past 15 years, she has been on hormone replacement therapy. She was surprised when I told her she needed to stop. I explained to her that hormone replacement therapy could put her at increased risk of a heart attack or stroke. Having placed her trust in one gynecologist for almost 20 years, Lori was hesitant to listen to my recommendation but said I could speak to her gynecologist. I did, and although he was aware of both of these studies, he insisted that he was able to watch Lori closely to make sure there were no untoward effects.

When Lori returned to my office one month later, she felt reassured that her gynecologist would be able to "watch her closely" to make sure that she would not be in danger. I pointed out that realistically, there is no situation in which patients are watched more closely than in a clinical trial; medical staff are constantly observing patients. In that setting, women were still dying and having strokes. Would you be willing to let your doctor watch you closely as you have a heart attack or a stroke? Neither was Lori. I saw her last month and she reports that there is a sense of relief now that she understands how high her risk was, and also that she feels no symptoms since stopping the medicine.

Kim was also upset when I recommended that she stop her hormone replacement therapy. At 52, Kim is overweight with mildly abnormal cholesterol. This was the reason she was started on hormone replacement therapy, prior to menopause, to help with her cholesterol levels (although HRT lowers cholesterol levels only slightly). That was eight years ago. Kim was resistant to stopping her hormone replacement therapy, as was her primary doctor. We decided to initiate therapy with a statin that would reduce her cholesterol optimally and thereby prove that the hormone replacement therapy was no longer necessary.

One month after starting statin therapy, a surveillance blood test revealed very slight irritation of the liver. We stopped the statin and a short time later initiated therapy with a second statin, which did not affect her liver and lowered her LDL to optimal levels (70s). At this point, I was able to convince both Kim and her doctor that the risks of HRT far outweighed the benefits, and she stopped it. Over the next six months, Kim has reported no significant difference in how she has felt since stopping her hormone replacement therapy. She also admitted that she was surprised to find that she had been taking a medicine all along that increased her risk of a heart attack or stroke, and was pleased that she did not need to take it any more.

Women: The Reality of Your Risk

- Be your own best advocate and insist on being treated aggressively. Focus on your own health and your major risks. Heart disease is the greatest danger you will face.
- "Borderline" blood pressure or "satisfactory" cholesterol levels put you at increased risk of a heart attack, stroke, or premature death.

- Make sure your blood pressure is less than 115 and your LDL is less than 100. The benefits are even greater by adopting a healthy lifestyle.

- If you develop symptoms of chest pain, shortness of breath, nausea or a change in exercise capacity that seem unusual for you, you need to call your doctor and determine whether you may be experiencing signs of a heart attack. The first symptom that you develop may not be the classic chest pain or pressure.

- You can achieve your health goals by using these established medicines with proven safety records that are the cornerstones of this plan: aspirin, statins, beta-blockers and ACE inhibitors.

- Put simply, be selfish and live longer.

PART 4

Commonsense Lifestyle Strategies

CHAPTER 16

Reducing Stress

WE ALL FEEL STRESSED. THE PACE OF LIFE HAS INCREASED, and some of the things that were invented to make our lives more convenient have simply made it more hectic. Consider technology—it has increased the speed with which we communicate, and as a result, there is now widespread demand for immediate responses. Fax, email, pagers, cell phones—where can a person hide for a half hour to relax?

While occasionally someone decides to turn life on its ear and take a six-month work sabbatical or even just an extended vacation, most of us can't afford that luxury. It's important to know the very real toll stress takes on your body. If you understand some of the physiology of it, you may have more respect for that tightness in your neck, your headache, your back pain, or your inability to sleep, and then be able to change your lifestyle even a little.

The Cardiovascular Effects of Stress

Stress can cause heart attacks and sudden death, primarily through the release of the stress hormones adrenaline and cortisol. Both hormones have important roles in helping us survive stressful situations, which was especially useful when humans were the hunted and not just the hunters.

Cortisol stimulates the release of sugar into the blood, providing an energy source for muscles and vital organs that can be metabolized quickly. It's primarily released in the morning, just prior to the time when you wake up. Adrenaline gives added energy under stress and is generally released when you're nervous or frightened—when you experience what is called the "fight or flight" response. In addition to serving the purposes for which they are needed, the release of stress hormones can cause several negative occurrences within the body.

Clot formation: The release of stress hormones causes certain blood cells (platelets) to become stickier and more prone to forming blood clots, which can lead to a heart attack or a stroke. That's why heart attacks are particularly likely to occur in the early hours of the day (when cortisol and adrenaline are released), or when we've just had an experience that "really stresses us out" (releasing adrenaline).

Arrhythmias: For the most part, arrhythmias are unpredictable, but natural disasters (earthquakes, hurricanes, etc.) do seem to trigger life-threatening arrhythmias, and it is thought that the stress hormones play a role in causing this to happen. Within the last decade, two reports have established the connection between arrhythmias and major crises. In the early 90s researchers documented that there was an increased risk of heart attacks and death in the first two days after a major California earthquake. People already diagnosed with heart disease had a significantly increased risk of life threatening arrhythmias during the first month after the World Trade Center disaster.

Direct effect on vascular system: The stress hormones make the muscle cells in the walls of the arteries contract, transiently narrowing the vessels and creating higher blood pressure. Even though this may be a relatively short-term effect, it is a potent stimulus for the muscle cells in the walls of the arteries to hypertrophy (grow abnormally larger), the way the muscles in your body will hypertrophy when you lift weights. This leads to structural changes in the arteries (they become thicker and stiffer) that lead to persistent elevation in blood pressure. When your blood pressure rises, this puts a great deal of additional stress on the heart.

Stress on the heart: As we've discussed throughout the book, when your vascular system becomes stiffer, the heart must work harder to push the blood through the arteries. Over a period of months or years, the extra workload damages the heart. Even when people develop what is called "white coat hypertension," transient high blood pressure that occurs primarily when being examined by a doctor (hence the reference to a "white coat"), the heart is damaged over time, signifying an increased risk for you. For decades doctors thought that transient increases in blood pressure were not a major concern, but now we know better.

Immune system dysfunction: Stress affects the immune system, causing changes within the blood vessels. As you remember from Chapter 2, the immune system's response plays a role in fighting off the fat and cholesterol that can become deposited on the walls of the arteries. If the immune system is compromised, this can shift this delicate balance to one in which the immune system can no longer perform its protective duties.

If you feel excessive stress, either constantly or intermittently, your heart and cardiovascular system are undergoing changes in addition to those caused by high cholesterol or high blood pressure, putting you at a much higher risk.

The Symptoms of Stress

Even after describing to patients all the terrible things stress does to their bodies, most people don't really do much about it. After all, you can't see or feel your vessels stiffen up, and you don't really know your heart is working harder, so it's tough to feel much urgency about the problem.

You may not realize how many symptoms of stress you have. If I talk to patients about the symptoms associated with high levels of stress, I can really get them talking: Are you tired all the time? Do you eat when you're not hungry? (This symptom can reflect impulsive behavior, related to stress.) Do you snap at family members without cause? Symptoms that are commonly experienced by people under stress include:

- Fatigue
- Anger
- Impatience
- More likely to smoke
- More likely to "slack off"
- Poor sleep
- Loss of focus
- Impulsive behavior

Although stress is not the most likely reason for all of these problems; it can be the cause.

Strategies

Unfortunately, there is no cure for stress. Instead, a series of steps can be taken to relieve you of stressful stimuli and improve your ability to cope with the stress that you face.

Identify your major stressors.

What are the major sources of your stress? Are things rocky at work? Do you have an ill relative? Is money tight? Is it as simple as the problem of surviving your morning commute? Are your kids at an age where the family has no downtime because of baseball, soccer, piano lessons and karate? List the things that bother you. Once you have specified what they are, you'll find it easier to either eliminate them or take them in stride.

Prioritize.

What is most important to you? Make a list of the "must have" ingredients of your life. Stress must not come between you and what you love most. Once you have recognized your priorities, you can take one of two approaches to stress:

Eliminate the stressor. If the situation that is causing stress isn't that important to you, begin an elimination process. Maybe you took on an optional committee responsibility at work or a volunteer job in your personal life that is not fulfilling anymore or is taking up too much time. At work, you might be able to delegate the work or get the job reassigned. With a volunteer commitment, you could resign or find someone else to fill the slot.

Accept what you cannot change. If the stress is caused by your job or a family member, obviously you're not going to be able to drop out of the scene and give up these responsibilities. Simply by identifying how much stress a situation is causing, you can sometimes reduce some of the negative feelings that are resulting from it.

Make an attitude adjustment.

Instead of hoping to eliminate or alter certain situations, try embracing the idea of change. For example, if you feel your job is in jeopardy for economic reasons, not for job performance reasons, that's stressful. Instead of losing sleep over something you can't control, start planning now for the logistics and finances to be in place so that you can withstand any potential job turmoil or transition.

Put yourself first at least once a day.

Start and end the day in a way you enjoy—or find a time in the middle of the day to call your own. In my case, I like to start my day before anybody else wakes up. I can enjoy the quiet of the sunrise and look out my window and watch the deer eat all of our perennials. I have more difficulty ending the day right; I have to race to get home and have dinner, find out how my kids' days were, help with their homework, and help put them to bed.

You need to figure out the key factors that will make your life better. Whether it's yoga or golf or sitting and reading a good book for 20 minutes, remember that if you don't make yourself a priority, no one else will.

Exercise.

Exercise is a great stress reducer. (Chapter 17 discusses exercise in more detail.) Think of exercise as a training opportunity. The same hormones are released with the same vascular effects as when you are under emotional stress. The body learns how to cope with these physiological changes in a way that makes the emotional stress better tolerated. While you may think that feeling "stressed out" gives your body plenty of training, the training gained during exercise is far better. Exercise provides a gradual buildup in the level of stress, a period of equilibrium during sustained activity, and a gradual reduction in stress during the cooldown period.

This prepares your body for the stress that you may experience at other times, making it easier for your body and psyche to respond and avoid a shock from the stress.

Eat well.

This may be the toughest component of a stress reduction program. Perhaps you are running from one task to another both at work and at home; eating breakfast in your car and lunch while working at your desk. Are dinners frequently a bite here and there after racing home from work? Whatever happened to a relaxed dinner with your family? I have friends who made a commitment years ago to go out to dinner every Thursday night, without their kids. This is a great approach; it contributes to eating right and definitely helps with stress.

Dealing with stress is much tougher than simply taking a few medications to extend your life, which is the main focus of this plan. The key to reducing stressful situations and their impact on your heart is to change both your attitude and your daily habits—tough tasks, but crucial ones.

CHAPTER 17

Adding Exercise

REMEMBER WHEN YOU USED TO JUMP AT THE CHANCE TO take a long walk, toss a ball, or ride a bicycle? What ever happen to that urge to be active, now that we really need it?

Patients consistently report that they have a greater sense of well being and their quality of life seems better upon completion of a regular exercise routine (although it usually takes about three months before these positive benefits are noticed). And those are just the mental benefits. The physical benefits are well known: Exercise lowers your risk of heart disease; it improves your metabolism; and weight loss decreases your risk of developing diabetes. In addition, weight-bearing exercise strengthens your bones (of particular importance in those of you at risk for osteoporosis). What's not to like?

Making the Commitment

In an ideal world, we would exercise daily. For most people, this is hard to do, and the toughest part about exercising is making the commitment to change your daily routine. When are you are going to exercise? Will you wake up earlier? Stay up later? If you're like most people, you find it difficult to exercise at work or in the middle of all your other daily activities. Sometimes it just seems that there is simply not room in your schedule, even though there needs to be.

Stacey is in her early 40s and has a strong family history of coronary artery disease, as her father underwent bypass surgery in his 60s. She is a busy executive with three children, and though she knows she needs to exercise to improve her health, she's found it difficult to fit an exercise routine into her daily life. When we talked, it became clear that Stacey was expecting too much of herself. She was trying to go from not exercising at all to exercising daily. While this is an admirable goal, it isn't very practical given that up until now exercise has not figured into her schedule at all.

I suggested that she start small. After thinking about it for a few minutes, Stacey started figuring out that she could exercise one week-day and both weekend days, enabling her to start a three-times-a-week routine—a major improvement over a zero-times-a-week program. Instead of trying to change her entire lifestyle, she could alter her schedule on one working day and exercise on the weekends. Hopefully, she will enjoy the routine and will eventually commit to exercising four or five days a week.

The Ideal Exercise Routine

Ideally, your exercise routine should be performed daily and consist of at least 30 minutes of aerobic activity. A proper routine starts with an appropriate warm-up and ends with a cool-down period. This program should consist of both stretching and resistive exercise training in order to build flexibility and strength of individual mus-cle groups.

Start with 5 minutes of warming up, then 20 minutes of aerobic activity, and finally 5 more minutes of a cool-down. By adding more stretching before and after, you lessen the risk of injury. Gradually increase the period of aerobic activity to 30 minutes, then, as you can manage, increase the intensity.

You may want to join a gym, enlist a personal trainer to get you started, or purchase a book on exercise. You might also consider the "buddy" system. You really will get out for that morning walk or run if you know someone else is going to do it with you.

If you already have heart disease (have suffered a heart attack or had an angioplasty or bypass operation), or even if you're over 40 and have not exercised for some time, you need to talk to your doctor before undertaking a new regimen. In all likelihood, your doctor will recommend that you undergo a maximal stress test to make sure you will be safe when you start exercising.

The Practical Approach to Exercise

Let's be practical. I know how hard it is to start a new routine, so I'm going to give you some guidance for a relatively easy way to get started—simply by becoming more active. Your goal should be a gradual increase in your activity to the point where you are getting aerobic exercise for 20 to 30 minutes at a time, in addition to warm-up and cool-down periods.

Most doctors don't recommend a specific exercise routine, as this is not something that many doctors have been taught to do, so here is a general framework for starting your plan:

Add more activity. If you were to burn only 15 calories more each day, you could prevent the weight gain that is so common in middle age. Park a block further from work or take the stairs instead of the elevator.

Pick the right activity for you. If jogging makes your knees hurt and your new house is too far from the indoor pool where you used to swim, select something new. The activity needs to be one that you are likely to enjoy, because without enjoyment there is no chance that you would continue with this activity long-term. For me, the ideal exercise is to play basketball, but at this point, having suffered through several orthopedic injuries, pounding around on a basketball court is just not workable for me. Similarly, people with osteoarthritis or other forms of arthritis are unlikely to become committed runners because of the stress that places on already compromised joints.

Consider your locale and the weather. Those who live in regions of extreme heat or extreme cold need to select activities that they can continue even during the winter and summer months, perhaps choosing separate ones for the indoor and outdoor seasons.

Be cautious during weather extremes. We've all heard about people, particularly those in southern states, who die mowing their lawns on a hot day in the middle of the summer. When they are taken to the hospital, their body temperature can be as high as 107 or 108. Every winter people die shoveling snow.

Consider any personal needs or limitations. If you have osteoporosis, you need an activity with significant weight bearing to add that stimulus to your body to strengthen your bones.

Establish a regular schedule for exercising. If exercise becomes part of your routine, just as natural as brushing your teeth, you'll find it easier to maintain an exercise program. And while the ideal goal is to exercise every day, and the minimum recommendation is three times a week, even exercising once a week is better than no activity. Getting out and being active a few times per week may not be enough to get out you into competitive shape, and it may or may not be enough to help you lose an extra 10 pounds, but it is likely to make you feel better and potentially even help you deal with stress a little bit more effectively.

Start your program slowly. Let's suppose that walking a block makes you very short of breath. Then the first day try walking that block slowly, picking up the pace a bit—or lengthening the walk—when you try it again the next day. The goal is to move as slowly as you need to so that you can eventually continue your activity for 30 minutes minimum without stopping. Once you have been able to continue your activity for 30 minutes, you will then be able to pick up the pace and increase the challenge. Once you can walk slowly for 30 minutes, you will gradually begin to increase your pace by walking more quickly for the last three to five minutes. Over time, you will lengthen the amount of your exercise at the faster pace until the entire 30 minutes is at that quicker pace. At that point you will attempt to increase the pace further, starting at the end of your routine.

Remember to warm up and cool down. Another component of starting slowly is warming up. There are many routines that people recommend for warm-ups, but a general rule is that five minutes of warm-up will be enough if you do not feel stiff and you do feel ready. At that point, start exercising slowly to make sure that you have warmed up enough.

Keep yourself hydrated. People tend to think that after a moderate exercise session their body needs sugar and potassium in addition to sodium and water. The truth is that very few of us need intense electrolyte or glucose replacement at the end of exercise. What we need most is water, and most of us would do best if we were drinking water throughout our exercise. If you have a medical problem that requires you to take a diuretic on a regular basis, you should discuss with your doctor how to judge how much water you need. It is easy to tell when you are not drinking enough water, because you feel lightheaded or washed out at the end of the routine. It also may be appropriate to ask your doctor whether you should skip your diuretic or take half a dose of diuretic on those days when you are exercising and it is warmer out. Your doctor will help you customize your medicines and your fluid intake based on your medical situation.

Keep your expectations realistic. Perhaps the most important part of an exercise routine is creating expectations that are realistic. Whenever you start an exercise routine, you will notice breathlessness, fatigue, and even muscle pains as you start to push your body harder. It is generally not considered a pleasant part of exercise. It typically takes a couple of months before you stop having these unpleasant effects of exercise, and it may take even longer if you are exercising less than three times a week.

I remember the summer that I first started running. The first two months were miserable, but I knew it was important to improve my overall cardiovascular condition. By the time fall came and the temperature turned colder, I was addicted to running. After you reach a stage of fitness, your body starts to release chemicals called endorphins during exercise, which affects your brain in a way that makes the experience a pleasant one. Since I am not a neuropharmacologist

I cannot explain it further, but I can tell you that it is well recognized both in the scientific and the fitness communities that the release of endorphins is responsible for the "runner's high." Once I got to that point, not even cold weather stopped me; I was outside running in my shorts and perhaps a sweatshirt—having a great time.

Exercise will make you feel better, and will reduce your risk of heart disease. If you choose the activity that's right for you, set up a schedule that you can keep, and use your common sense to gradually increase the intensity of the routine as your body can handle, you will start to feel better within the first few weeks. As you plan your exercise program, you can feel confident in knowing that your risks can be reduced even before you put on your running shoes for the first time by having implemented the Before It Happens Plan.

CHAPTER 18

The Heart-Healthy Eating Plan

THERE ARE TWO THINGS I WON'T DO IN THIS CHAPTER. I WILL not tell you about a new diet plan to help you lose weight. I also won't tell you to lose weight (although it would improve your health in the long run). The purpose of my eating plan is to make sure you don't sabotage the tremendous benefit of the Before It Happens Plan by eating yourself to death.

Many times I have started a patient on a statin only to find that three months later, after dropping total cholesterol under 160 and LDL below 80, these wonderful effects seemed to be interpreted as "steak insurance," leading to a major increase of meat in the diet. (Yes, you can have a bit more fat in your diet after treatment with a statin, but you still need to pay attention.)

As a cardiologist, I understand the potential benefit of good nutrition. But with patient after patient unable or unwilling to follow the ideal diet, my approach evolved to accept that people usually can't change their diets very much. As I completed a presentation at a hospital's grand rounds, I was stopped by an offended internist. She couldn't believe I had spent almost my entire presentation discussing the use of these four medicines to prevent death and disability, while only acknowledging the role of lifestyle in one sentence. I agreed with her concern and tried to reassure her that the plan provides maximum impact. Although she did not seem satisfied, I did check her plate at the lunch that followed. Be assured, she may not favor my approach with these medicines, but she also doesn't follow a healthy diet.

Considering human nature as well as the experience in my practice, I believe that the best philosophy to follow is this: *Eat less, avoid processed foods and follow a well-balanced diet.*

Eating less is contrary to everything around us, restaurants with all-you-can-eat menus, super-sized drinks and side orders at fast food chains. I stopped to get a cup of coffee on a recent trip, and there were no coffee cups that fit into my car's cup holders (in 1996, when my car was made, we still drank 12 ounces of coffee at a time, not 16 or 24 ounces).

> We eat until we are full, instead of eating until we are no longer hungry.

The next time you eat out, see how many people finish their entrées. Almost everyone—and that's in addition to an appetizer and a dessert for many. Do you routinely get seconds when eating dinner at home? I know it tastes good, but there needs to be a limit. I know this is not so easy, so let me explain a few ways to curb your appetite.

Some Excellent Diet Plans and the Art of Eating Less

Simply eating less would make you healthier, but most people are happiest with some type of "plan" for changing their eating habits. For that reason, I'm going to recommend that you pick up a copy of either *The South Beach Diet* or one of Dean Ornish's books.

One of the things I like about Dr. Agatston's *The South Beach Diet* is that it focuses largely on the concept that the more processed food you eat, the more likely you are to eat more processed food. The book reviews the studies that prove that highly processed carbohydrates make us crave even more of those carbohydrates. The author's approach is successful because he focuses the reader on a diet that takes away the unhealthy foods that encourage unhealthy eating. You can eat carbohydrates and fats, you just can't eat the ones that are really bad. Yes, it is a diet to lose weight, but it really is a diet for healthier eating.

Similarly, Dr. Ornish's program focuses on improved health, not weight loss. In fact, the diet is only part of Ornish's approach to a comprehensive change in lifestyle. Ornish's diet relies on plant protein and avoids animal proteins. Like Agatston, Ornish also focuses on complex carbohydrates and avoiding processed foods, reducing your hunger.

In contrast, Dr. Atkins's diet leads to significant weight loss by shifting metabolism to a mode called ketosis. Although some studies suggest that certain individuals may note improvement in their cholesterol profile in addition to weight loss, many patients will see their LDL level increase dramatically, a correlate of increased risk for a heart attack or stroke. On the positive side, the Atkins diet addresses the problem of overeating. By eating protein and fat, and no carbohydrates, your appetite for carbohydrates disappears and you eat less.

Other Diet Plans: The Well-Balanced Diet

The South Beach Diet and the Ornish program both recommend a nutritionally balanced diet. Both programs provide for appropriate protein and complex carbohydrates, and both seem to provide adequate fat (although the Ornish diet includes much less). In both of these programs, the type of fats and carbohydrates are key. Saturated fat is bad, so replacing it with unsaturated fat will help, as long as you don't use more unsaturated fat than the amount of saturated fat you had been using.

Other diets will also provide a well-balanced and nutritionally sound option, including the Mediterranean diet and the DASH program from the American Heart Association. In all cases, success car-

---

Control your urge to overeat by:

- Drinking water
- Eating more frequently, so you don't become ravenous
- Eating carbohydrates with a low glycemic index
- Reducing stress

ries a common thread: eat less, avoid simple and processed carbohydrates (with a high glycemic index) and balance protein, fat and carbohydrates.

The Mediterranean diet refers to a diet rich in monounsaturated fats, a type of fat that provides a significant proportion of the daily caloric intake but does not affect cholesterol. The diet is high in fruits, vegetables, nuts and seeds, with dairy products and beans as the primary protein sources (minimal red meat). Wine is an important part of the diet.

Interest in the diet stems from the low rates of heart disease in Mediterranean countries, although that could be partially explained by lifestyle or genetic factors. The American Heart Association points out on their website that this diet can worsen obesity due to its high proportion of calories from fats.

In the early 1990s, a group of investigators created a diet that seemed to promise a food-related way to control blood pressure. It became known as the DASH diet, after the name of the initial study called the Dietary Approaches to Stop Hypertension. The study showed that over an 8-week period, the diet reduced blood pressure. (Although they were not compared directly in a study, the impact of the DASH diet on blood pressure is much less than the effects that would be anticipated from the medicines in the Before It Happens Plan.)

The DASH diet stresses fruits, vegetables and low-fat dairy foods. It is a high-fiber diet with low saturated and total fat content. The diet features foods rich in potassium, calcium and magnesium. If you were to look at the plan, you would see that it seems similar to the Ornish and South Beach diets, although there are some obvious differences. The National Institutes of Health sponsored the DASH studies, so the information about the studies and the diet is available online in the section titled "Information for Patients" at http://www.nhlbi.nih.gov/ guidelines/hypertension/index.htm.

Practically speaking, if you could reduce your calories by as little as 10 percent daily, you would see the benefits within 2 to 3 months. All of the benefits of a healthier diet and weight loss are complementary to the medicines in the Before It Happens Plan. To truly minimize your risks, you need both, but whether or not you can change, the Before It Happens Plan *will* reduce your risks of heart attack, stroke or premature death.

CHAPTER 19

Conclusion:
Don't Worry about the Costs,
Just Keep Your Family Alive

CONSISTENTLY, DOCTORS RAISE ONE CONCERN ABOUT THE
Before It Happens program. It isn't its safety. It isn't doubt about its
scientific basis. It's the cost. I admit it, this plan will be costly to society, but it will provide more tangible benefits than most investments
our country makes. Besides, if you can afford it, these medicines are
an investment that has a wonderful return—keeping you alive.

A few months ago, I bought more life insurance. It turns out that
the insurance company considered me worthy of their best rates—
$1,650 for a million-dollar policy. Then I realized that, although I was
buying life insurance, what I really wanted was life assurance, some
way to make sure I stayed alive.

The Before It Happens Plan is life assurance. This value can be
expressed in terms of the personal financial cost. If you had no prescription drug coverage, and needed all four medicines, the cost
would range from $1,225 to $2,925 yearly, depending upon whether
you took all generics or the best-studied brands. That's not much different than my annual premium for life insurance. If you have prescription coverage as part of your health insurance, your personal cost
would be only a few hundred dollars a year. (If not, see if your
employer offers the option.) The Before It Happens Plan becomes
much more affordable.

The Test of Confidence: What about My Family?

My wife told me the most revealing question she asks her doctors: "Would you give your wife these medicines?" This is the quintessential question in addressing safety. So here's what happens in my house. My wife's risk is very low, based on the test results listed in the following chart.

	My Wife	Me
Age	45	42
Blood Pressure	110/70	112/68
Total Cholesterol	166	153
HDL Cholesterol	53	60
LDL Cholesterol	98	85
Smoker?	No	No
Diabetes?	No	No
Family History of concern	Mother	No
Body Mass Index (Should be < 25)	21	25
Activity	Exercises regularly	Exercises intermittently

But here's where numbers can be deceiving. My mother-in-law died suddenly last year from heart disease. She was 69, and she didn't seem to be at risk either. I had recently asked her to check on her test results. Her blood pressure was under 115/75 and her LDL was less than 100. Although she took an aspirin a day, she also took hormone replacement therapy, and had for years. While on vacation, she suddenly died of a heart attack.

According to standard teaching, her age of 69 at the time of her death means that this does not signify any increase in risk for my wife. But this view misses the point of the concept of risk. Yes it would be more significant if it had happened when my mother-in-law were 49, but it signifies a possibility of risk for my wife. Based on recent studies, it is possible that my mother-in-law's heart attack could also have been due to her hormone replacement therapy.

In either case, I view this as a risk factor, and here is the plan for my wife (which she actually agrees to). When she hits 50, or as soon as she begins to enter menopause, she will start on a statin. I wouldn't try an ACE inhibitor or beta-blocker because she has taken medicines in the past that lowered blood pressure only slightly but made her very dizzy. As she completes menopause, she will start on 81 mg a day of aspirin.

At 45, I will start on my baby aspirin. Considering that my blood pressure always used to be under 105/60, I expect that I will be on an ACE inhibitor, too, since it will likely reach the 120s by then. (Studies show that 90 percent of us who reach 50 without being diagnosed with high blood pressure go on to develop it in subse quent years.)

Studies show that the strategies of my program reduce the risk of cardiovascular disease, and do so safely. That's why I am so comfortable "prescribing" this program to my family and myself.

People Want to Take Medicines That Reduce Risk

You aren't the only one willing to take medicines that can keep you alive. Most people talk about how they resent having to take medicines, but when asked, almost everyone is willing. A recent survey by CNN.com asked whether people would be willing to take medicines every day to prevent heart attacks and strokes; 94 percent said yes.

Help your family and friends get what they want: medicines to keep them alive and healthy.

You Have the Power

The Before It Happens Plan is simple, safe and effective. Best of all, you have taken control of your health and guided your doctor to treat you optimally. Now look around at your family and friends. They could become another statistic, unless you save their lives.

With over half of American adults having a blood pressure above 115//75 and half having an LDL above 100, the risk surrounds you. Just go up to your family and friends, one at a time or all at once. Tell them this.

- "I just read a book that explained why I was at risk of a heart attack, stroke or dying young, and it showed me how to take control of my health to save my life. It wasn't hard."
- "The book showed me how high our risks really are, and I am worried about your risk. Take this book, and call me if you need any help with it."

I've got to tell you, there is no greater rush that you can feel than when you save a life. You have that same power now.

Warning Signs of Heart Trouble

In the movies, people who have heart attacks clutch their chests as if in pain and keel over. This isn't necessarily how it happens in real life. Many heart attacks start slowly; you may feel a mild pain, sick to your stomach, or just generally uncomfortable—you may not even be sure what is wrong. Sometimes symptoms come and go. To make it even more complicated, symptoms differ for men and for women and can change from one heart attack to another. When my grandfather had his first heart attack, he felt chest pressure, but with his second, nausea and vomiting.

However, if you know the general signs of heart attack and what steps to take in an emergency, you may be able to save a life—even your own.

Warning Signs for Men

Chest discomfort. The feeling of discomfort may range from uncomfortable pressure on the chest to a feeling like squeezing or outright pain. Most times the pain is near the center of the chest and usually lasts for more than a few minutes. However, it can also subside and then return again.

Other types of upper body discomfort. Some people experience pain in the back, neck, jaw or stomach, and sometimes the pain will be in one or both arms.

Shortness of breath. This may occur before the chest discomfort, but it often comes along with the chest pain. Diabetics are more likely to have shortness of breath without chest pain than non-diabetics, so the textbooks say. However, unexplained shortness of breath should always lead to a conversation with your doctor, and if it doesn't resolve after resting a few minutes, a call to 9-1-1 would be prudent.

Nausea, lightheadedness, or unexplained sweating. These other symptoms can also sometimes signal a heart attack.

Warning Signs for Women

Female heart attack victims tend to be about 10 years older than men, so women sometimes think they have less to worry about than their male counterparts. This isn't true. Tragically, women are much less likely to think that any discomfort they feel might be attributed to a heart attack, and as a result, they often don't seek help in time. Women currently account for nearly half of all heart attack deaths.

As for men, chest discomfort is often the first symptom to present itself in women, but women are more likely to experience nausea, shortness of breath, or lightheadedness as early signs, so all these symptoms need to be taken seriously.

Here is a brief rundown of symptoms for women:

- Pain or discomfort in the center of the chest, classically described as pressure
- Nausea
- Shortness of breath
- Lightheadedness
- Breaking out in a cold sweat
- Pain or discomfort in other areas of the upper body including arms, back, neck, jaw or stomach
- Reduction in exercise capacity; tiring easily

For Men and Women

Here's what to do if you experience any of the above symptoms:

- If pain is severe, call 9-1-1 right away. Moments count.
- If symptoms are mild or confusing, wait five minutes (no longer!); if the symptoms are still present call 9-1-1. It's better to be sent home with a diagnosis of "heartburn" than to find that you or a loved one were actually trying to "tough out" a heart attack.

Life-Saving Measures to the Rescue

> Remember, once you have a heart attack or stroke, the damage cannot be reversed—not with this plan or any other.

Once you're in an ambulance or reach the hospital, there are many measures that can be taken to save your life. You may need clot-busting drugs or artery-opening treatments, both of which can stop a heart attack in progress. However, you need this help immediately. *An hour after your first symptom may be too late.*

Studies show that most heart attack victims wait two hours or more after their symptoms begin before they seek medical help. (Women, minorities, and the elderly are the most likely to delay seeking help, feeling that "it will go away.") This delay can result in death or damage to the heart that can cause lifelong disability.

If you're hesitant to call 9-1-1 and instead assume a family member can drive you to the hospital, think again. Studies show that heart attack victims who arrive by ambulance benefit doubly—procedures can be started by the emergency medical service (EMS) workers on board the ambulance. Most carry defibrillators (equipment that restarts the heart if beating has stopped), nitroglycerin, morphine, and oxygen, all of which can be helpful in an emergency. In addition, many ambulance companies relay a patient's medical condition to the hospital prior to arrival, meaning that the emergency room staff knows what to do the moment the person arrives. Patients who arrive by ambulance also receive faster medical care.

Some people have heard that popping an aspirin is the thing to do if they think they are having a heart attack. Don't take the time to even think about this or look for the aspirin, just call 9-1-1. The EMS team who arrives may give an aspirin, but by that time, you're under medical care, and these pros have a wide arsenal of tools at their disposal to save your life.

Plan Ahead

You've implemented the plan and reduced your risk. But the risk can never be zero (death is unavoidable, but it is postponable). If you live in a major city, you can consider which hospital provides the best care. It's not just a matter of finding out how the local paper rates them, but also how their emergency room is staffed, if cardiologists are on call and if they have the ability to perform an emergency angioplasty within an hour of you entering the emergency room, if indeed you are having a heart attack. If two hospitals are equally situated, the one with

---

What Doctors Need to Know about You in an Emergency:

Create an index card for each member of the family noting:

- All health conditions you have or have had (asthma, thyroid condition, heart murmur etc.)
- All medicines you take
- Any medicines to which you are allergic

The card should also include:

- Your doctor's telephone number (day and on-call, if the numbers are different)
- The name and number of the person to contact if you are taken to the hospital

cardiologists on call who can perform emergency angioplasty is preferable. Of course, an ambulance may not give you a choice.

Next, you need to write down vital health information that any doctor treating you for anything would need to know.

Take care of these things now—it really can make a life-or-death difference.

What to Do If You Think You're Having a Heart Attack

At the beginning of a heart attack, you need to act quickly. Almost a third of people die suddenly during their heart attack, before they can even call for help. You can't take this lightly. Call 9-1-1, sit down and use your nitroglycerin under your tongue (ask your doctor about this).

Interpreting Test Results

To individualize the plan to your needs, a series of standard tests needs to be performed. The only risk of these tests is the possibility of a lax interpretation of the results. If you ever look at a report of one of your tests, whether it be a blood test, stress test or any other medical test, you will notice that normal ranges are listed next to your results. It would seem that the interpretation is simple, within the normal range is good, outside of it is bad. But that is not necessarily true.

Normal ranges are defined based upon the purpose of performing the test. As an illustration, I will show you the actual data for the BNP blood test, along with the ways that normal ranges could be selected based on the way the test is to be used.

Figure B.1 helps explain the statistical limitations of defining the normal range. These data show how a blood test can be used to figure out whether heart disease is the cause of the symptom of shortness of breath. The actual data from the study are plotted, and I have added the dotted lines marked A, B, C and D. The way the graph works is this: The boxes exclude those people whose test results were in the lowest or highest quartile, while the lines that extend above and below the boxes show the limits of the most extreme values. If the highest normal value were selected to be at the line marked A everyone who had shortness of breath caused by heart disease would be correctly identified, since even the lower edge of the bar on the right is above

Diagnostic Testing; Normal Ranges

Using a Blood Test to
Diagnose the Reason
for Shortness of Breath

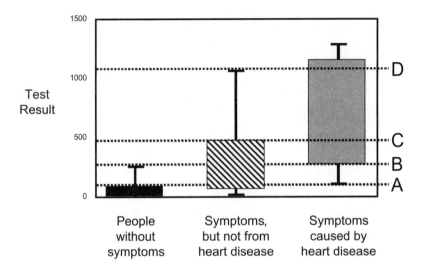

Figure B.1 This graph shows the importance of defining the normal range for a diagnostic blood test.

As described in the text, moving the highest normal value from line A to line D changes the meaning of the test result. At A, the test detects everyone with heart disease (gray group), but about 25 percent of normal people with no symptoms and no heart disease are told that there is a problem (black group). (After a period of anxiety, further tests would prove they don't need to worry about that test result.)

If C were used, some people with heart disease would be incorrectly told that they don't require treatment, when in fact they do, but some people with the same symptom caused by another disease (striped group) would be told they need treatment for heart disease, when in fact they wouldn't.

Without understanding what you are trying to learn from performing a test, results such as these can create more anxiety and confusion than anything else.

A. However, that means that almost a quarter of people who had no symptoms and no heart disease would have an abnormal test. This particular test is one for an advanced type of heart disease that can be as dangerous as many kinds of cancer. Imagine feeling fine, walking in to your doctor, getting this test done, then being told (erroneously) that you had a heart condition that could kill you within five years. To avoid this situation, it would be better if B were used as the cutoff for abnormal, since everyone who was normal has a result below B.

In clinical practice, this test is used to learn whether the symptom of shortness of breath is caused by your heart or by something else, and either C or D could be used to make the distinction. You can see that neither is perfect. C incorrectly identifies 25 percent of people with symptoms but without heart disease as having heart disease while missing about 40 percent with it. D won't label anyone erroneously as having heart disease, but will identify less than a third of patients with it.

Without considering these pitfalls, the interpretation of tests becomes a crap-shoot.

Selection of a threshold either includes too many people without the problem, or fails to find enough people with it. Similarly, treatment plans either include more people than is absolutely necessary or leave some in need of a therapy unprotected. Because the medicines in this program are so safe—safer than most vitamins—and save lives, I prefer to treat a few extra people to make sure that one more person doesn't suffer or die unnecessarily. The standard guidelines rest on the premise that my preference, and this plan, is too costly. But I think you are worth the extra cost.

Appendix C

Insurance Issues

Insurance companies try to keep their costs as low as possible, but they won't refuse to pay for necessary medical care unless they specify those limitations explicitly in your policy. That doesn't mean they won't try to avoid a bill. That's why they generally require approval in advance for more expensive tests and treatments. Sometimes you will need to get approval; sometimes your doctor will need to ask. Never assume anyone else has taken care of this for you; always call your insurance company before the test or treatment and confirm the medical services are covered and ask for the authorization number (and any limitations).

Your goal is to make it easy for your insurance company to say yes. To do so, ask in advance whenever possible (they may call this pre-certification or authorization). The only part of the Before It Happens program that may require discussion with an insurance company is the performance of an echocardiogram. But even this test should be simple to get your company to pay for. Many doctors seem concerned that an insurance company will not cover an echocardiogram and the patients will be "stuck" with the bill. In fact, this is unlikely to happen.

The standard treatment guidelines recommend an echocardiogram when there is a suspicion of heart failure. That's all the professional organizations require—a suspicion. That should be enough for your insurance company, but you should call to make sure. Tell them that your doctor suspects you have heart failure and ask them if an echocardiogram is a test that is covered by your plan. (They will say yes, if your doctor considers it medically necessary.) Then ask if any special paperwork or precertification is required for the test. (They will probably say no.) Then remind your doctor to write on the insurance forms and medical records that the test is being performed to make sure that you don't have heart failure.

It is possible that your doctor did not suspect heart failure, so you will explain why you are concerned, and this will raise your doctor's suspicion. According to the American Heart Association and the American College of Cardiology, anyone who has been diagnosed with coronary artery disease or who has high blood pressure, high cholesterol or diabetes is at risk of heart failure. That means your doctor should suspect it, so that is what you should tell your doctor is the reason that you want the echocardiogram. If you don't have any of these conditions, look at Figure 2.2 in Chapter 2; you probably have coronary artery disease and just don't feel it yet.

If your doctor still seems resistant, show him or her the graph below. All doctors know that the risk of colon cancer is real, and typically people get tested at age 50. The incidence of people having heart failure (an advanced form of heart disease) is much higher than the risk of colon cancer. Heart failure is at least as dangerous, more common and would warrant specific treatment. Show this to your doctor, and get him or her to order an echocardiogram.

Life Insurance

As you start the Before It Happens Plan, ask yourself one more question. In addition to this life assurance plan, do I need more life insurance? If you do, get the insurance first. The life insurance companies make sure you are healthy according to the standard guidelines, and having a blood pressure of 134/83 is not worrisome to them, so you can still get your new policy at a reasonable price. Once you start taking medicines, you will pay significantly more for your life insurance. Insurance, then assurance—that needs to be your plan.

Your Doctor Will Tell You to Get Tested for Colon Cancer. Advanced Heart Failure Is More Common (and More Dangerous)

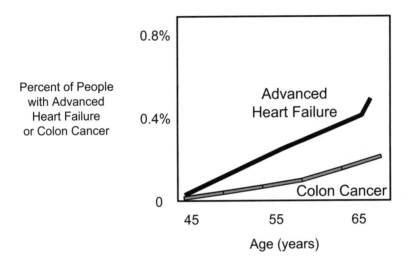

Figure C.1 Doctors are supposed to tell everyone to be tested for colon cancer, and with good reasons. This deadly disease is easy to diagnose and treat when a regular routine of colonoscopies is followed.

People with advanced heart failure are at even higher risk of death and disability than people diagnosed with colon cancer. According to data from the National Cancer Institute and the Framingham Study, heart failure, an advanced form of heart disease, is much more common than colon cancer in young people, and becomes even more so as people age.

A simple ultrasound of your heart can determine if you have the early changes in your heart structure indicating you are at risk of advanced heart failure. If that were the case, the medicines of the Before It Happens Plan could prevent you from getting sick or dying.

Prescription Medicines for Heart Disease

The medicines commonly used for the treatment of cardiovascular disease are listed here, including those integral to the Before It Happens Plan (statins, beta-blockers and ACE inhibitors), those that may be necessary to add (diuretics, ARBs) and those that should be used only for specific situations (calcium channel blockers).

Generic Name	Brand Name
Statins	
atorvastatin	Lipitor
fluvastatin	Lescol, Lescol XL
lovastatin	Mevacor, Altocor
pravastatin	Pravachol
rosuvastatin	Crestor
simvastatin	Zocor
Beta-Blockers	
acebutolol	Sectral
atenolol	Tenormin
betaxolol	Kerlone
bisoprolol	Zebeta

Generic Name	Brand Name
carteolol	Cartrol
carvedilol	Coreg
labetolol	Normodyne, Trandate
metoprolol succinate	Toprol-XL
metoprolol tartrate	Lopressor
nadolol	Corgard
pindolol	Visken
propranolol	Inderal
timolol	Blocadren

ACE Inhibitors

benazepril	Lotensin
captopril	Capoten
enalapril	Vasotec
fosinopril	Monopril
lisinopril	Prinivil, Zestril
moexipril	Univasc
perindopril	Aceon
quinapril	Accupril
ramipril	Altace
trandolapril	Mavik

Angiotensin Receptor Antagonists

candesartan	Atacand
eprosartan	Teveten
irbesarten	Avapro
losartan	Cozaar
olmesartan	Benicar
telmisartan	Micardis
valsartan	Diovan

Generic Name	Brand Name

Diuretics

amiloride	Midamar
amiloride +	
hydrochlorothiazide	Moduretic
chlorthalidone	Hygroton
furosemide	Lasix
hydrochlorothiazide	Esidrix, Hydrodiuril,
	Microzide
indapamide	Lozol
metolazone	Mykrox, Zaroxolyn
spironolactone	Aldactone
spironolactone +	
hydrochlorothiazide	Aldactazide
triamterene	Dyrenium
triamterene +	
hydrochlorothiazide	Dyazide, Maxzide

Calcium Channel Blockers

amlodipine	Norvasc
bepridil	Vascor
diltiazem	Cardizem CD,
	Cardizem SR,
	Dilacor XR, Tiazac
felodipine	Plendil
isradipine	DynaCirc, DynaCirc CR
nicardipine	Cardene SR
nifedipine	Adalat CC, Procardia XL
nimodipine	Nimotop
nisoldipine	Sular
verapamil	Calan SR, Covera HS,
	Isoptin SR, Verelan

Selected Bibliography

Statistics on Cardiovascular Disease

American Heart Association. (2003) *Epidemiology of CV Disease, Heart Disease and Stroke Statistics—2003 Update.* Vol. 2003. American Heart Association.

Medicines

Beta-Blockers

Beta Blocker Heart Attack Trial Research Group. (1982). A randomized trial of propranolol in patients with acute myocardial infarction. I. Mortality results. *Journal of the American Medical Association, 247,* 1707–1714. [Source for Figure 4.3]

Bristow, M. R., Gilbert, E. M., Abraham, W. T., et al. (1996). Carvedilol produces dose-related improvements in left ventricular function and survival in subjects with chronic heart failure. *Circulation, 94,* 2807–2816. [Source for Figure 4.3]

CIBIS-II investigators and Committee (1999). The Cardiac Insufficiency Bisoprolol Study II (CIBIS-II): a randomised trial. *Lancet, 353,* 9–13.

Dargie, H. J. (2001). Effect of carvedilol on outcome after myocardial infarction in patients with left-ventricular dysfunction: The CAPRICORN randomised trial. *Lancet, 357,* 1385–1390.

Gottlieb, S. S., McCarter, R. J., & Vogel, R. A. (1998). Effect of beta-blockade on mortality among high-risk and low-risk patients after myocardial infarction. *New England Journal of Medicine, 339,* 489–497.

Hjalmarson, A., Elmfeldt, D., Herlitz, J., et al. (1981). Effect on mortality of metoprolol in acute myocardial infarction: A double-blind randomised trial. *Lancet, 2,* 823–827.

MERIT-HF Study Group. (1999). Effect of metoprolol CR/XL in chronic heart failure: Metoprolol CR/XL Randomised Intervention Trial in Congestive Heart Failure (MERIT-HF). *Lancet, 353,* 2001–2007. [Source for Figure 4.3]

Norwegian Multicenter Study Group. (1981). Timolol-induced reduction in mortality and reinfarction in patients surviving acute myocardial infarction. *New England Journal of Medicine, 304,* 801–807.

Olsson, G., Tuomilehto, J., Berglund, G., et al. (1991). Primary prevention of sudden cardiovascular death in hypertensive patients: Mortality results from the MAPHY Study. *American Journal of Hypertension, 4,* 151–158. [Source for Figure 4.3]

Packer, M., Coats, A. J., Fowler, M. B., et al. (2001). Effect of carvedilol on survival in severe chronic heart failure. *New England Journal of Medicine,* 344, 1651–1658. [Source for Figure 4.3]

Packer, M., Colucci, W. S., Sackner-Bernstein, J. D., et al., for the PRECISE study group. (1996). Double-blind, placebo-controlled study of the effects of carvedilol in patients with moderate to severe heart failure. *Circulation, 94,* 2793–2799. [Source for Figure 4.3]

Poole-Wilson, P. A., Swedberg, K., Cleland, J. G., et al. (2003). Comparison of carvedilol and metoprolol on clinical outcomes in patients with chronic heart failure in the Carvedilol Or Metoprolol European Trial (COMET): Randomised controlled trial. *Lancet, 362,* 7–13.

Sackner Bernstein, J. D., & Mancini, D. M. (1995). Rationale for treatment of patients with chronic heart failure with adrenergic blockade. *Journal of the American Medical Association, 274,* 1462–1467.

Wikstrand, J., Warnold, I., Olsson, G., Tuomilehto, J., Elmfeldt, D., & Berglund, G. (1988). Primary prevention with metoprolol in patients with hypertension: Mortality results from the MAPHY study. *Journal of the American Medical Association, 259,* 1976–1982.

Yancy, C. W., Fowler, M. B., Colucci, W. S., et al. (2001). Race and the response to adrenergic blockade with carvedilol in patients with chronic heart failure. *New England Journal of Medicine, 344,* 1358–1365.

Aspirin

Cleland, J. G. (2002). Is aspirin "the weakest link" in cardiovascular prophylaxis? The surprising lack of evidence supporting the use of aspirin for cardiovascular disease. *Progress in Cardiovascular Disease, 44,* 275–292.

Cyrus, T., Sung, S., Zhao, L., Funk, C. D., Tang, S., & Pratico, D. (2002, September 3). Effect of low-dose aspirin on vascular inflammation, plaque stability, and atherogenesis in low-density lipoprotein receptor-deficient mice. *Circulation, 106*(10), 1282–1287.

Department of Health and Human Services Food and Drug Administration, 21 CFR Part 343 [Docket No. 77N–094A] RIN 0910–AA01. (1998, October 23). Internal Analgesic, Antipyretic, and Antirheumatic Drug Products for Over-the-Counter Human Use: Final Rule for Professional Labeling of Aspirin, Buffered Aspirin, and Aspirin in Combination with Antacid Drug Products. Federal Register, Vol. 63, No. 205, Rules and Regulations. Available at http://www.fda.gov/ohrms/dockets/98fr/102398c.pdf

FDA/Center for Drug Evaluation and Research. (n.d.). Before Using Aspirin to Lower Your Risk of Heart Attack or Stroke, Here Is What You Should Know: Only a health professional can safely decide if the regular use of aspirin to prevent a heart attack or stroke is right for you. Last updated March 13, 2003, at http://www.fda.gov/cder/consumerinfo/AspirinFactSheet.pdf.

Hayden, M., Pignone, M., Phillips, C., & Mulrow, C. (2002, January 15). Aspirin for the primary prevention of cardiovascular events: A summary of the evidence for the U.S. Preventive Services Task Force. *Annals of Internal Medicine, 136*(2), 161–172. Summary for patients in *Annals of Internal Medicine, 136*(2), I55.

Second International Study of Infarct Survival Collaborative Group. (1988). Randomised trial of intravenous streptokinase, oral aspirin, both, or neither among 17,187 cases of suspected acute myocardial infarction: ISIS-2. *Lancet, 2,* 349–360.

U.S. Preventive Services Task Force. (2002, January 15) Aspirin for the primary prevention of cardiovascular events: Recommendation and rationale. *Annals of Internal Medicine, 136*(2), 157–160.

ACE Inhibitors

Acute Infarction Ramipril Efficacy (AIRE) Study Investigators. (1993). Effect of ramipril on mortality and morbidity of survivors of acute myocardial infarction with clinical evidence of heart failure. *Lancet, 342,* 821–828.

Anderson, T. J., Elstein, E., Haber, H., & Charbonneau, F. (2000). Comparative study of ACE-inhibition, angiotensin II antagonism, and calcium channel blockade on flow-mediated vasodilation in patients with coronary disease (BANFF study). *Journal of the American College of Cardiology, 35,* 60–66.

CONSENSUS Trial Study Group. (1987). Effects of enalapril on mortality in severe congestive heart failure: Results of the Cooperative North Scandinavian Enalapril Study. *New England Journal of Medicine, 316,* 1429–1435.

Estacio, R. O., Jeffers, B. W., Hiatt, W. R., Biggerstaff, S. L., Gifford, N., & Schrier, R. W. (1998, March 5). The effect of nisoldipine as compared with enalapril on cardiovascular outcomes in patients with non-insulin-dependent diabetes and hypertension. *New England Journal of Medicine, 338*(10), 645–652.

Hirsch, A. T., Talsness, C. E., Schunkert, H., Paul, M., & Dzau, V. J. (1991). Tissue-specific activation of cardiac angiotensin converting enzyme in experimental heart failure. *Circulation Research, 69,* 475–482.

ISIS-4 (Fourth International Study of Infarct Survival) Collaborative Group. (1995). ISIS-4: A randomised factorial trial assessing early oral captopril, oral mononitrate, and intravenous magnesium sulphate in 58,050 patients with suspected acute myocardial infarction. *Lancet, 345,* 669–685.

Kjoller-Hansen, L., Steffensen, R., & Grande, P. (2000, March 15). The Angiotensin-converting Enzyme Inhibition Post Revascularization Study (APRES). *Journal of the American College of Cardiology, 35*(4), 881–888.

Kober, L., Torp-Pedersen, C., Carlsen, J. E., et al. (1995). A clinical trial of the angiotensin-converting-enzyme inhibitor trandolapril in patients with left ventricular dysfunction after myocardial infarction. Trandolapril Cardiac Evaluation (TRACE) Study Group. *New England Journal of Medicine, 333,* 1670–1676.

Lewis, E. J., Hunsicker, L. G., Bain, R. P., & Rohde, R. D. (1993). The effect of angiotensin-converting-enzyme inhibition on diabetic nephropathy. The Collaborative Study Group. *New England Journal of Medicine, 329,* 1456–1462.

Mancini, G. B., Henry, G. C., Macaya, C., et al. (1996). Angiotensin-converting enzyme inhibition with quinapril improves endothelial vasomotor dysfunction in patients with coronary artery disease. The TREND (Trial on Reversing ENdothelial Dysfunction) Study. *Circulation, 94,* 258–265.

Oosterga, M., Voors, A. A., Pinto, Y. M., Buikema, H., Grandjean, J. G., Kingma, J. H., Crijns, H. J., & van Gilst, W. H. (2001, March 1). Effects of quinapril on clinical outcome after coronary artery bypass grafting (The QUO VADIS Study): QUinapril on Vascular Ace and Determinants of Ischemia. *American Journal of Cardiology, 87*(5), 542–546.

Pfeffer, M. A., Braunwald, E., Moye, L. A., et al. (1992). Effect of captopril on mortality and morbidity in patients with left ventricular dysfunction after myocardial infarction: Results of the survival and ventricular enlargement trial. *New England Journal of Medicine, 327,* 669–677.

Pitt, B., Poole-Wilson, P. A., Segal, R., et al. (2000). Effect of losartan compared with captopril on mortality in patients with symptomatic heart failure: Randomised trial—the Losartan Heart Failure Survival Study ELITE II. *Lancet, 355,* 1582–1587.

Pitt, B., Segal, R., Martinez, F. A., et al. (1997). Randomised trial of losartan versus captopril in patients over 65 with heart failure (Evaluation of Losartan in the Elderly Study, ELITE). *Lancet, 349,* 747–752.

Scholkens, B. A., & Landgraf, W. (2002). ACE inhibition and atherogenesis. *Canadian Journal of Physiology and Pharmacology, 80,* 354–359.

SOLVD Investigators. (1991). Effect of enalapril on survival in patients with reduced left ventricular ejection fractions and congestive heart failure. *New England Journal of Medicine, 325,* 293–302.

SOLVD Investigators. (1992). Effect of enalapril on mortality and the development of heart failure in asymptomatic patients with reduced left ventricular ejection fractions. *New England Journal of Medicine, 327,* 685–691.

Tatti, P., Pahor, M., Byington, R. P., Di Mauro, P., Guarisco, R., Strollo, G., & Strollo, F. (1998, April 21). Outcome results of the Fosinopril versus Amlodipine Cardiovascular Events Randomized Trial (FACET) in patients with hypertension and NIDDM. *Diabetes Care, 21*(4), 597–603.

Wright, J.T., Jr., Bakris, G., Greene, T., Agodoa, L. Y., Appel, L. J., Charleston, J., Cheek, D., Douglas-Baltimore, J. G., Gassman, J., Glassock, R., Heber,t L., Jamerson, K., Lewis, J., Phillips, R. A., Toto, R. D., Middleton, J. P., & Rostand, S. G.; African American Study of Kidney Disease and Hypertension Study Group. (2002, November 20). Effect of blood pressure lowering and antihypertensive drug class on progression of hypertensive kidney disease: Results from the AASK trial. *Journal of the American Medical Association, 288*(19), 2421–2431.

Yusuf, S., Sleight, P., Pogue, J., Bosch, J., Davies, R., & Dagenais, G. (2000). Effects of an angiotensin-converting-enzyme inhibitor, ramipril, on cardiovascular events in high-risk patients. The Heart Outcomes Prevention Evaluation Study Investigators. *New England Journal of Medicine, 342,* 145–153.

Statins

Brown, B. G., Zhao, X. Q., Chait, A., Fisher, L. D., Cheung, M. C., Morse, J. S., Dowdy, A. A., Marino, E. K., Bolson, E. L., Alaupovic, P., Frohlich, J., & Albers, J. J. (2002, November 29). Simvastatin and niacin, antioxidant vitamins, or the combination for the prevention of coronary disease. *New England Journal of Medicine, 345*(22), 1583–1592. Summary for patients in *Current Cardiology Reports* 4(6), 486.

Chilton, R., & O'Rourke, R. A. (2001, December). The expanding role of HMG-CoA reductase inhibitors (statins) in the prevention and treatment of ischemic heart disease. *Current Problems in Cardiology, 26*(12), 734–764.

Collins, R., Armitage, J., Parish, S., Sleigh, P., & Peto, R. (2003). MRC/BHF Heart Protection Study of cholesterol-lowering with simvastatin in 5,963 people with diabetes: A randomised placebo-controlled trial. *Lancet, 361,* 2005–2016. [Source for Figure 4.1]

Downs, J. R., Clearfield, M., Weis, S., Whitney, E., Shapiro, D. R., Beere, P. A., Langendorfer, A., Stein, E. A., Kruyer, W., & Gotto, A. M., Jr. (1998, May 27).

Primary prevention of acute coronary events with lovastatin in men and women with average cholesterol levels: Results of AFCAPS/TexCAPS. Air Force/Texas Coronary Atherosclerosis Prevention Study. *Journal of the American Medical Association, 279*(20), 1615–1622.

Heart Protection Study Collaborative Group. (2002). MRC/BHF Heart Protection Study of cholesterol lowering with simvastatin in 20,536 high-risk individuals: A randomised placebo-controlled trial. *Lancet,* 360, 7–22. [Source for Figure 4.1]

Long-Term Intervention with Pravastatin in Ischaemic Disease (LIPID) Study Group. (1998). Prevention of cardiovascular events and death with pravastatin in patients with coronary heart disease and a broad range of initial cholesterol levels. *New England Journal of Medicine, 339,* 1349–1357. [Source for Figure 4.1]

Pfeffer, M. A., Keech, A., Sacks, F. M., Cobbe, S. M., Tonkin, A., Byington, R. P., Davis, B. R., Friedman, C. P., & Braunwald, E. (2002, May 21). Safety and tolerability of pravastatin in long-term clinical trials: Prospective Pravastatin Pooling (PPP) Project. *Circulation, 105*(20), 2341–2346.

Pitt, B., Waters, D., Brown, W. V., van Boven, A. J., Schwartz, L, Title, L. M., Eisenberg, D., Shurzinske, L., & McCormick, L. S. (1999, July 8). Aggressive lipid-lowering therapy compared with angioplasty in stable coronary artery disease. Atorvastatin versus Revascularization Treatment Investigators. *New England Journal of Medicine, 341*(2), 70–76.

Sacks, F. M., Pfeffer, M. A., Moye, L. A., et al. (1996). The effect of pravastatin on coronary events after myocardial infarction in patients with average cholesterol levels. Cholesterol and Recurrent Events Trial investigators. *New England Journal of Medicine, 335,* 1001–1009. [Source for Figure 4.1]

Scandinavian Simvastatin Survival Study Group. (1994). Randomised trial of cholesterol lowering in 4444 patients with coronary heart disease: The Scandinavian Simvastatin Survival Study (4S). *Lancet, 344,* 1383–1389. [Source for Figure 8.1]

Schwartz, G. G., Olsson, A. G., Ezekowitz, M. D., Ganz, P., Oliver, M. F., Waters, D., Zeiher, A., Chaitman, B. R., Leslie, S., & Stern, T.; Myocardial Ischemia Reduction with Aggressive Cholesterol Lowering (MIRACL) Study Investigators. (2001, April 4).Effects of atorvastatin on early recurrent ischemic events in acute coronary syndromes: The MIRACL study: a randomized controlled trial. *Journal of the American Medical Association, 285*(13), 1711–1718. [Source for Figure 4.1]

Sever, P. S., Dahlof, B., Poulter, N. R., Wedel, H., Beevers, G., Caulfield, M., Collins, R., Kjeldsen, S. E., Kristinsson, A., McInnes, G. T., Mehlsen, J., Nieminen, M., O'Brien, E., & Ostergren, J.; ASCOT investigators. (2003, April 5). Prevention of coronary and stroke events with atorvastatin in hypertensive patients who have average or lower-than-average cholesterol concentrations, in the Anglo-Scandinavian Cardiac Outcomes Trial—Lipid Lowering Arm (ASCOT-LLA): A multicentre randomised controlled trial. *Lancet, 361*(9364), 1149–1158.

Shepherd, J., Cobbe, S. M., Ford, I., Isles, C. G., Lorimer, A. R., MacFarlane, P. W., McKillop, J. H., & Packard, C. J. (1995, November 16). Prevention of coronary heart disease with pravastatin in men with hypercholesterolemia. West of Scotland Coronary Prevention Study Group. *New England Journal of Medicine, 333*(20), 1301–1307.

Velasco, J. A. (1999). After 4S, CARE and LIPID—Is evidence-based medicine being practised? *Atherosclerosis, 147*(Supplement 1), S39–S44.

ARBs

Brenner, B. M., Cooper, M. E., de Zeeuw, D., et al. (2001). Effects of losartan on renal and cardiovascular outcomes in patients with type 2 diabetes and nephropathy. *New England Journal of Medicine, 345,* 861–869.

Cohn, J. N., & Tognoni, G. (2001). A randomized trial of the angiotensin-receptor blocker valsartan in chronic heart failure. *New England Journal of Medicine, 345*(23), 1667–1675.

Lewis, E. J. (2002). The role of angiotensin II receptor blockers in preventing the progression of renal disease in patients with type 2 diabetes. *American Journal of Hypertension, 10,* 123S–128S.

Lewis, E. J., Hunsicker, L. G., Clarke, W. R., et al. (2001). Renoprotective effect of the angiotensin-receptor antagonist irbesartan in patients with nephropathy due to type 2 diabetes. *New England Journal of Medicine, 345,* 851–860.

Pfeffer, M. A., Swedberg, K., Granger , C. B., et al. (2003). Effects of candesartan on mortality and morbidity in patients with chronic heart failure: The CHARM-Overall programme. *Lancet, 362,* 759–766.

Sasso, F. C., Carbonara, O., Persico, M., et al. (2002). Irbesartan reduces the albumin excretion rate in microalbuminuric type 2 diabetic patients independently of hypertension: A randomized double-blind placebo-controlled crossover study. *Diabetes Care, 25,* 1909–1913.

Diuretics

ALLHAT Officers and Coordinators for the ALLHAT Collaborative Research Group. (2002, December 18). Major outcomes in high-risk hypertensive patients randomized to angiotensin-converting enzyme inhibitor or calcium channel blocker vs. diuretic: The Antihypertensive and Lipid-Lowering Treatment to Prevent Heart Attack Trial (ALLHAT). *Journal of the American Medical Association, 288*(23), 2981–2997.

Weinberger, M. H. (1992). Mechanisms of diuretic effects on carbohydrate tolerance, insulin sensitivity and lipid levels. European Heart Journal, 13(Supplement G), 5–9.

Calcium Blockers

Packer, M., O'Connor, C. M., Ghali, J. K., et al. (1996). Effect of amlodipine on morbidity and mortality in severe chronic heart failure. Prospective Randomized Amlodipine Survival Evaluation Study Group. *New England Journal of Medicine, 335,* 1107–1114.

Pahor, M., Psaty, B. M., Alderman, M. H., Applegate, W. B., Williamson, J. D., Cavazzini, C., & Furberg, C. D. (2000, December 9). Health outcomes associated with calcium antagonists compared with other first-line antihypertensive therapies: A meta-analysis of randomised controlled trials. *Lancet, 356*(9246), 1949–1954.

Vitamins

Liem, A., Reynierse-Buitenwerf, G. H., Zwinderman, A. H., Jukema, J. W., & van Veldhuisen, D. J. (2003, June 18). Secondary prevention with folic acid: effects on clinical outcomes. *Journal of the American College of Cardiology, 41*(12), 2105–2113.

Morris, C. D., & Carson, S. (2003, July 1). Routine vitamin supplementation to prevent cardiovascular disease: A summary of the evidence for the U.S. Preventive Services Task Force. *Annals of Internal Medicine, 139*(1), 56–70.

Schnyder, G., Roffi, M., Pin, R., Flammer, Y., Lange, H., Eberli, F. R., Meier, B., Turi, Z. G., & Hess, O. M. (2001, November 29). Decreased rate of coronary restenosis after lowering of plasma homocysteine levels. *New England Journal of Medicine, 345*(22), 1593–1600.

U.S. Preventive Services Task Force. (2003, July 1). Routine vitamin supplementation to prevent cancer and cardiovascular disease: Recommendations and rationale. *Annals of Internal Medicine, 139*(1), 51–55.

U.S. Preventive Services Task Force. (2003, July 1). Summaries for patients. Taking vitamin supplements to prevent cardiovascular disease and cancer: Recommendations from the U.S. Preventive Services Task Force. *Annals of Internal Medicine, 139*(1), I–76.

Vivekananthan, D. P., Penn, M. S., Sapp, S. K., Hsu, A., & Topol, E. J. (2003, June 14). Use of antioxidant vitamins for the prevention of cardiovascular disease: Meta-analysis of randomised trials. *Lancet, 361*(9374), 2017–2023.

Yusuf, S., Dagenais, G., Pogue, J., Bosch, J., & Sleight, P. (2000). Vitamin E supplementation and cardiovascular events in high-risk patients. The Heart Outcomes Prevention Evaluation Study Investigators. *New England Journal of Medicine, 342*, 154–160.

Lifestyle

Appel, L. J., Champagne, C. M., Harsha, D. W., Cooper, L. S., Obarzanek, E., Elmer, P. J., Stevens, V. J., Vollmer, W. M., Lin, P. H., Svetkey, L. P., Stedman, S. W., & Young, D. R.; Writing Group of the PREMIER Collaborative Research Group. (2003, April 23–30). Effects of comprehensive lifestyle modification on blood pressure control: Main results of the PREMIER clinical trial. *Journal of the American Medical Association, 289*(16), 2083–2093.

Appel, L. J., Moore, T. J., Obarzanek, E., Vollmer, W. M., Svetkey, L. P., Sacks, F. M., Bray, G. A., Vogt, T. M., Cutler, J. A., Windhauser, M. M., Lin, P. H., & Karanja, N.)1997, April 17). A clinical trial of the effects of dietary patterns on blood pressure. DASH Collaborative Research Group. *New England Journal of Medicine, 336*(16), 1117–1124.

Ezzati, M., Hoorn, S. V., Rodgers, A., Lopez, A. D., Mathers, C. D., & Murray, C. J.; Comparative Risk Assessment Collaborating Group. (2003, July 26). Estimates of global and regional potential health gains from reducing multiple major risk factors. *Lancet, 362*(9380), 271–280.

Ornish, D., Scherwitz, L. W., Billings, J. H., Brown, S. E., Gould, K. L., Merritt, T. A., Sparler, S., Armstrong, W. T., Ports, T. A., Kirkeeide, R. L., Hogeboom, C., & Brand, R. J. (1998, December, 16). Intensive lifestyle changes for reversal of coronary heart disease. *Journal of the American Medical Association, 280*(23), 2001–2007.

Sacks, F. M., Svetkey, L. P., Vollmer, W. M., Appel, L. J., Bray, G. A., Harsha, D., Obarzanek, E., Conlin, P. R., Miller, E. R., 3rd, Simons-Morton, D. G., Karanja, N., & Lin, P. H.; DASH-Sodium Collaborative Research Group. (2001, January 4). Effects on blood pressure of reduced dietary sodium and the Dietary Approaches to Stop Hypertension (DASH) diet. *New England Journal of Medicine, 344*(1), 3–10.

Sebregts, E. H., Falger, P. R., & Bar, F. W. (2000, April-May). Risk factor modification through nonpharmacological interventions in patients with coronary heart disease. Journal of Psychosomatic Research, 48(4–5), 425–441.

Guidelines for Management

Chobanian, A. V., Bakris, G. L., Black, H. R., et al. (2003). The Seventh Report of the Joint National Committee on Prevention, Detection, Evaluation, and Treatment of High Blood Pressure: The JNC 7 Report. Journal of the American Medical Association, 289, 2560–2571.

Gordon, A. J., & Macpherson, D. S. (2003, June 1). Guideline chaos: Conflicting recommendations for preoperative cardiac assessment. American Journal of Cardiology, 91(11), 1299–1303.

National Institutes of Health. (2002). Third Report of the Expert Panel on Detection, Evaluation, and Treatment of High Blood Cholesterol in Adults (Adult Treatment Panel III) Full Report. Vol. 2003. Available at http://www.nhlbi.nih.gov/guidelines/cholesterol/index.htm

Sackner-Bernstein, J. (2003). The JNC 7 hypertension guidelines. Journal of the American Medical Association, 290, 1312.

Sackner-Bernstein, J. (in press). Why are the JNC-7 targets different from the evidence? [Letter to the editor]. Journal of the American Medical Association.

Woolf, S. H. (1999, December 22–29). The need for perspective in evidence-based medicine. Journal of the American Medical Association, 282(24), 2358–2365.

Characteristics or Conditions

Diabetes

Adler, A. I., Stratton, I. M., Neil, H. A., et al. (2000). Association of systolic blood pressure with macrovascular and microvascular complications of type 2 diabetes (UKPDS 36): Prospective observational study. British Medical Journal, 321, 412–419.

American Diabetes Association. (2003). National Diabetes Fact Sheet. Vol. 2003.

Balkau, B., Shipley, M., Jarrett, R. J., Pyorala, K., Pyorala, M., Forhan, A., & Eschwege, E. (1998, March). High blood glucose concentration is a risk factor for mortality in middle-aged nondiabetic men. 20-year follow-up in the Whitehall Study, the Paris Prospective Study, and the Helsinki Policemen Study. Diabetes Care, 21(3), 360–367.

Diabetes Control and Complications Trial/Epidemiology of Diabetes Interventions and Complications Research Group. (2002, February 10). Retinopathy and nephropathy in patients with type 1 diabetes four years after a trial of intensive therapy. New England Journal of Medicine, 342(6), 381–389.

Garvey, W. T., & Hermayer, K. L. (1998). Clinical implications of the insulin resistance syndrome. Clinical Cornerstone, 1, 13–28.

Giugliano, D., Acampora, R., Marfella, R., et al. (1997). Metabolic and cardiovascular effects of carvedilol and atenolol in non-insulin-dependent diabetes mellitus and hypertension: A randomized, controlled trial. Annals of Internal Medicine, 126, 955–959.

Haffner, S. M. (1999). Epidemiology of insulin resistance and its relation to coronary artery disease. *American Journal of Cardiology, 84,* 11J–14J.

Khaw, K-T., Wareham, N., Luben, R., et al. (2001). Glycated haemoglobin, diabetes, and mortality in men in Norfolk cohort of European Prospective Investigation of Cancer and Nutrition (EPIC-Norfolk). *British Medical Journal, 322,* 1–6. [Source for Figure 10.1]

McGill, H. C., Jr., McMahan, C. A., Malcom, G. T., Oalmann, M. C., & Strong, J. P. (1995, April). Relation of glycohemoglobin and adiposity to atherosclerosis in youth. Pathobiological Determinants of Atherosclerosis in Youth (PDAY) Research Group. *Arteriosclerosis, Thrombosis, and Vascular Biology,.15*(4), 431–440.

Pontiroli, A. E., Pacchioni, M., Camisasca, R., & Lattanzio, R. (1998). Markers of insulin resistance are associated with cardiovascular morbidity and predict overall mortality in long-standing non-insulin-dependent diabetes mellitus. *ACTA Diabetologica, 35,* 52–56.

Raji, A., Seely, E. W., Bekins, S. A., Williams, G. H., & Simonson, D. C. (2003). Rosiglitazone improves insulin sensitivity and lowers blood pressure in hypertensive patients. *Diabetes Care, 26,* 172–178.

Reneland, R., Alvarez, E., Andersson, P. E., Haenni, A., Byberg, L., & Lithell, H. (2000). Induction of insulin resistance by beta-blockade but not ACE-inhibition: Long-term treatment with atenolol or trandolapril. *Journal of Human Hypertension, 14,* 175–180.

Saydah, S. H., Loria, C. M., Eberhardt, M. S., & Brancati, F. L. (2001, March). Subclinical states of glucose intolerance and risk of death in the U.S. *Diabetes Care, 24*(3), 447–453.

Shargorodsky, M., Wainstein, G., Gavish, E., et al. (2003). Treatment with rosiglitazone reduces hyperinsulinemia and improves arterial elasticity in patients with type 2 diabetes mellitus: Rosiglitazone improves insulin sensitivity and lowers blood pressure in hypertensive patients. *American Journal of Hypertension, 16,* 617–622.

Stratton, I. M., Adler, A. I., Neil, H. A., Matthews, D. R., Manley, S. E., Cull, C. A., Hadden, D., Turner, R. C., & Holman, R. R. (2000, August 12). Association of glycaemia with macrovascular and microvascular complications of type 2 diabetes (UKPDS 35): Prospective observational study. *British Medical Journal, 321*(7258), 405–412.

Torlone, E., Britta, M., Rambotti, A. M., et al. (1993). Improved insulin action and glycemic control after long-term angiotensin-converting enzyme inhibition in subjects with arterial hypertension and type II diabetes. *Diabetes Care, 16,* 1347–1355.

U.K. Prospective Diabetes Study Group. (1998, September 12). Efficacy of atenolol and captopril in reducing risk of macrovascular and microvascular complications in type 2 diabetes: UKPDS 39. *British Medical Journal, 317*(7160), 713–720.

Hypertension

Adler, A. I., Stratton, I. M., Neil, H. A., Yudkin, J. S., Matthews, D. R., Cull, C. A., Wright, A. D., Turner, R. C., & Holman, R. R. (2000, August 12). Association of systolic blood pressure with macrovascular and microvascular complications of type 2 diabetes (UKPDS 36): Prospective observational study. *British Medical Journal, 321*(7258), 412–419.

Hansson, L., Zanchetti, A., Carruthers, S. G., Dahlof, B., Elmfeldt, D., Julius, S., Menard, J., Rahn, K. H., Wedel, H., & Westerling, S. (1998, June 13). Effects of intensive blood-pressure lowering and low-dose aspirin in patients with hypertension: Principal results of the Hypertension Optimal Treatment (HOT) randomised trial. HOT Study Group. *Lancet, 351*(9118), 1755–1762.

Kannel, W. B. (1996). Cardioprotection and antihypertensive therapy: The key importance of addressing the associated coronary risk factors (the Framingham experience). *American Journal of Cardiology, 77,* 6B–11B.

Kannel, W. B. (2000). Elevated systolic blood pressure as a cardiovascular risk factor. *American Journal of Cardiology, 85,* 251–255.

Lewington, S., Clarke, R., Qizilbash, N., Peto, R., & Collins, R. (2002). Age-specific relevance of usual blood pressure to vascular mortality: A meta-analysis of individual data for one million adults in 61 prospective studies. *Lancet, 360,* 1903–1913. [Source for Figure 6.1]

Muscholl, M. W., Hense, H-W., Brockel, U., et al. (1998). Changes in left ventricular structure and function in patients with white coat hypertension: Cross sectional survey. *British Medical Journal, 317,* 565–570. [Source for Figure 7.2]

Plante, G. E. (1994). The blood vessel as a target organ in hypertension: protective effect of perindopril. *Canadian Journal of Cardiology, 10*(Supplement D), 25D–29D.

Pooling Project Research Group. (1978). Relationship of blood pressure, serum cholesterol, smoking habit, relative weight, and ECG abnormalities to incidence of major coronary events: Final Report of the Pooling Project. Journal of Chronic Diseases, 31, 201–306.

Seshadri, S., Wolf, P. A., Beiser, A., et al. (2001). Elevated midlife blood pressure increases stroke risk in elderly persons: The Framingham Study. *Archives of Internal Medicine, 161,* 2343–2350.

Vasan, R. S., Beiser, A., Seshadri, S., et al. (2002). Residual lifetime risk for developing hypertension in middle-aged women and men: The Framingham Heart Study. *Journal of the American Medical Association, 287,* 1003–1010. [Source for Figure 7.1]

Vasan, R. S., Larson, M. G., Leip, E. P., et al. (2001). Impact of high-normal blood pressure on the risk of cardiovascular disease. *New England Journal of Medicine, 345,* 1291–1297.

Wolf-Maier, K., Cooper, R. S., Banegas, J. R., Giampaoli, S., Hense, H. W., Joffres, M., Kastarinen, M., Poulter, N., Primatesta, P., Rodriguez-Artalejo, F., Stegmayr, B., Thamm, M., Tuomilehto, J., Vanuzzo, D., & Vescio, F. (2003, May 14). Hypertension prevalence and blood pressure levels in 6 European countries, Canada, and the United States. *Journal of the American Medical Association, 289*(18), 2363–2369.

Cholesterol and the Vessel Wall

De Franco, A. C., & Nissen, S. E. (2001). Coronary intravascular ultrasound: implications for understanding the development and potential regression of atherosclerosis. *American Journal of Cardiology, 88,* 7M–20M.

Dzau, V. J. (1993). Tissue renin-angiotensin system in myocardial hypertrophy and failure. *Archives of Internal Medicine, 153,* 937–942.

Kannel, W. B. (1995). Range of serum cholesterol values in the population developing coronary artery disease. *American Journal of Cardiology, 76,* 69C–77C.

Maseri, A., & Fuster, V. (2003, April 29). Is there a vulnerable plaque? *Circulation, 107*(16), 2068–2071.

McGill, H. C., Jr., McMahan, C. A., Herderick, E. E., Zieske, A. W., Malcom, G. T., Tracy, R. E., & Strong, J. P.; Pathobiological Determinants of Atherosclerosis in Youth (PDAY) Research Group. (2002, June 11). Obesity accelerates the progression of coronary atherosclerosis in young men. *Circulation, 105*(23), 2712–2718.

McGill, H. C., Jr., McMahan, C. A., Malcom, G. T., Oalmann, M. C., & Strong, J. P. (1997, January). Effects of serum lipoproteins and smoking on atherosclerosis in young men and women. The PDAY Research Group. *Arteriosclerosis, Thrombosis, and Vascular Biology, 17*(1):95–106.

McGill, H. C., Jr., McMahan, C. A., Zieske, A. W., Malcom, G. T., Tracy, R. E., & Strong, J. P. (2001, March 20). Effects of nonlipid risk factors on atherosclerosis in youth with a favorable lipoprotein profile. *Circulation, 103*(11), 1546–1550.

McGill, H. C., Jr., McMahan, C. A., Zieske, A. W., Sloop, G. D., Walcott, J. V., Troxclair, D. A., Malcom, G. T., Tracy, R. E., Oalmann, M. C., & Strong, J. P. (2000, August). Associations of coronary heart disease risk factors with the intermediate lesion of atherosclerosis in youth. The Pathobiological Determinants of Atherosclerosis in Youth (PDAY) Research Group. *Arteriosclerosis, Thrombosis, and Vascular Biology, 20*(8), 1998–2004.

McGill, H. C., Jr., McMahan, C. A., Zieske, A. W., Tracy, R. E., Malcom, G. T., Herderick, E. E., & Strong, J. P. (2000, July 25). Association of coronary heart disease risk factors with microscopic qualities of coronary atherosclerosis in youth. *Circulation, 102*(4), 374–379.

Nissen, S. E. (1999). Shortcomings of coronary angiography and their implications in clinical practice. *Cleveland Clinic Journal of Medicine, 66,* 479–485.

Nissen, S. E. (2000). Rationale for a post-intervention continuum of care: Insights from intravascular ultrasound. *American Journal of Cardiology, 86,* 12H–17H.

Nissen, S. E. (2002). Who is at risk for atherosclerotic disease? Lessons from intravascular ultrasound. *American Journal of Medicine, 112*(Supplement 8A), 27S–33S.

Rainwater, D. L., McMahan, C. A., Malcom, G. T., Scheer, W. D., Roheim, P. S., McGill, H. C., Jr., & Strong, J. P. (1999, March). Lipid and apolipoprotein predictors of atherosclerosis in youth: Apolipoprotein concentrations do not materially improve prediction of arterial lesions in PDAY subjects. The PDAY Research Group. *Arteriosclerosis, Thrombosis, and Vascular Biology, 19*(3), 753–761.

Sharrett, A. R., Ballantyne, C. M., Coady, S. A., et al., for the Atherosclerosis Risk in Communities Study Group. (2001). Coronary heart disease prediction from lipoprotein cholesterol levels, triglycerides, lipoprotein(a), apolipoproteins A-I and B, and HDL density subfractions: The Atherosclerosis Risk in Communities (ARIC) Study. *Circulation,* 104, 1108–1113. [Source for Figure 4.2]

Tuzcu, E. M., Kapadia, S. R., Tutar, E., et al. (2001). High prevalence of coronary atherosclerosis in asymptomatic teenagers and young adults: Evidence from intravascular ultrasound. *Circulation, 103,* 2705–2710. [Source for Figure 2.2]

Wilson, P. W., & Kannel, W. B. (1993). Hypercholesterolemia and coronary risk in the elderly: The Framingham Study. *American Journal of Geriatric Cardiology, 2,* 56.

Obesity

Kannel, W. B., Wilson, P. W., Nam, B. H., & D'Agostino, R. B. (2002). Risk stratification of obesity as a coronary risk factor. *American Journal of Cardiology, 90,* 697–701.

Kenchaiah, S., Evans, J. C., Levy, D., et al. (2002). Obesity and the risk of heart failure. *New England Journal of Medicine, 347,* 305–313.

Lee, M., Manson, J. E., Hennekens, C. H., & Paffenbarger, R. S. (1993). Body weight and mortality: A 27-year follow-up of middle-aged men. *Journal of the American Medical Association, 270,* 2823–2828.

Lew, E. A., & Garfinkel, L. (1979). Variations in mortality by weight among 750,000 men and women. *Journal of Chronic Diseases, 32,* 563–576. [Source for Figure 11.1]

McGill, H. C., Jr., McMahan, C. A., Herderick, E. E., Zieske, A. W., Malcom, G. T., Tracy, R. E., & Strong, J. P.; Pathobiological Determinants of Atherosclerosis in Youth (PDAY) Research Group. (2002, June 11). Obesity accelerates the progression of coronary atherosclerosis in young men. *Circulation, 105*(23), 2712–2718.

Willett, W. C., Manson, J. E., Stampfer, M. J., et al. (1995). Weight, weight change, and coronary heart disease in women: Risk within the normal weight range. *Journal of the American Medical Association, 273,* 461–465.

Women

Burke, A. P., Farb, A., Malcom, G. T., Liang, Y., Smialek, J., & Virmani, R. ((1998, June 2). Effect of risk factors on the mechanism of acute thrombosis and sudden coronary death in women. *Circulation, 97*(21), 2110–2116.

Hulley, S., Grady, D., Bush, T., Furberg, C., Herrington, D., Riggs, B., & Vittinghoff, E. (1998, August 19). Randomized trial of estrogen plus progestin for secondary prevention of coronary heart disease in postmenopausal women. Heart and Estrogen/progestin Replacement Study (HERS) Research Group. *Journal of the American Medical Association, 280*(7), 605–613.

Manson, J. E., Hsia, J., Johnson, K. C., Rossouw, J. E., Assaf, A. R., Lasser, N. L., Trevisan, M., Black, H. R., Heckbert, S. R., Detrano, R., Strickland, O. L., Wong, N. D., Crouse, J. R., Stein, E., & Cushman, M.; Women's Health Initiative Investigators. (2003, August 7). Estrogen plus progestin and the risk of coronary heart disease. *New England Journal of Medicine*349(6), 523–534.

Marcuccio, E., Loving, N., Bennett, S. K., & Hayes, S. N. (2003, January-February). A survey of attitudes and experiences of women with heart disease. *Womens Health Issues, 13*(1), 23–31.

Rapp, S. R., Espeland, M. A., Shumaker, S. A., Henderson, V. W., Brunner, R. L., Manson, J. E., Gass, M. L., Stefanick, M. L., Lane, D. S., Hays, J., Johnson, K. C., Coker, L. H., Dailey, M., & Bowen, D.; WHIMS Investigators. (2003, May 28). Effect of estrogen plus progestin on global cognitive function in postmenopausal women: The Women's Health Initiative Memory Study: A randomized controlled trial. *Journal of the American Medical Association, 289*(20), 2663–2672.

Shumaker, S. A., Legault, C., Thal, L., Wallace, R. B., Ockene, J. K., Hendrix, S. L., Jones, B. N., 3rd, Assaf, A. R., Jackson, R. D., Kotchen, J. M., Wassertheil-Smoller, S., & Wactawski-Wende, J.; WHIMS Investigators. (2003, May 28). Estrogen plus progestin and the incidence of dementia and mild cognitive impairment in postmenopausal women: The Women's Health Initiative Memory Study: A randomized controlled trial. *Journal of the American Medical Association, 289*(20), 2651–2662.

Stampfer, M. J., Hu, F. B., Manson, J. E., Rimm, E. B., & Willett, W. C. (2000, July 6). Primary prevention of coronary heart disease in women through diet and lifestyle. *New England Journal of Medicine, 343*(1), 16–22.

Wassertheil-Smoller, S., Hendrix, S. L., Limacher, M., Heiss, G., Kooperberg, C., Baird, A., Kotchen, T., Curb, J. D., Black, H., Rossouw, J. E., Aragaki, A., Safford, M., Stein, E., Laowattana, S., & Mysiw, W J.; WHI Investigators. (2003, May 28). Effect of estrogen plus progestin on stroke in postmenopausal women: The Women's Health Initiative: A randomized trial. *Journal of the American Medical Association, 289*(20), 2673–2684.

HIV

Bozzette, S. A., Ake, C. F., Tam, H. K., Change, S. W., & Louis, T. A. (2002). Cardiovascular and cerebrovascular events in patients treated for human immunodeficiency virus infection. *New England Journal of Medicine, 348,* 702–710.

Currier, J. S., Taylor, A., Boyd, F., Dezii, C. M., Kawabata, H., Burtcel, B., Maa, J. F., Hodder, S. (2003, August 1). Coronary heart disease in HIV-infected individuals. *Journal of Acquired Immune Deficiency Syndrome, 33*(4), 506–512.

David, M. H., Hornung, R., & Fichtenbaum, C. J. (2002, January 1). Ischemic cardiovascular disease in persons with human immunodeficiency virus infection. *Clinical Infectious Diseases, 34*(1), 98–102.

Grunfeld C., Kotler D.P., Hamadeh, R., Tierney, A,, Wang J., Pierson, RN. (1989). Hypertriglyceridemia in the acquired immunodeficiency syndrome. *American Journal of Medicine, 86,* 27–31.

Lenert, L. A., Feddersen, M., Sturley, A., & Lee, D. (2002). Adverse effects of medications and trade-offs between length of life and quality of life in human immunodeficiency virus infection. *American Journal of Medicine, 113,* 229–232.

Rebolledo, M. A., Krogstad, P., Chen, F., Shannon, K. M., & Klitzner, T. S. (1998). Infection of human fetal cardiac myocytes by a human immunodeficiency virus-1-derived vector. *Circulation Research, 83,* 738–742.

Sudden Death

Burke, A. P., Kolodgie, F. D., Farb, A., Weber, D. K., Malcom, G. T., Smialek, J., & Virmani, R. (2001, February 20). Healed plaque ruptures and sudden coronary death: Evidence that subclinical rupture has a role in plaque progression. *Circulation, 103*(7), 934–940.

Farb, A., Burke, A. P., Tang, A. L., Liang, T. Y., Mannan, P., Smialek, J., & Virmani, R. (1996, April 1). Coronary plaque erosion without rupture into a lipid core: A frequent cause of coronary thrombosis in sudden coronary death. *Circulation, 93*(7), 1354–1363.

Farb, A., Tang, A. L., Burke, A. P., Sessums, L., Liang, Y., & Virmani, R. (1995, October 1). Sudden coronary death. Frequency of active coronary lesions, inactive coronary lesions, and myocardial infarction. *Circulation, 92*(7), 1701–1709.

Kannel, W. B., Wilson, P. W., D'Agostino, R. B., & Cobb, J. (1998). Sudden coronary death in women. *American Heart Journal, 136,* 205–212.

Moss, A. J., Zareba, W., Hall, W. J., et al. (2002). Prophylactic implantation of a defibrillator in patients with myocardial infarction and reduced ejection fraction. *New England Journal of Medicine, 346,* 877–883.

Index

About the Author

Dr. Jonathan Sackner Bernstein is Director of Clinical Research at the Heart Failure Prevention and Treatment Clinic at the Heart Failure and Cardiomyopathy Center at North Shore University Hospital in Manhasset, New York. He has been published in *Circulation, Transplantation* and the *Journal of the American Medical Association*. He majored in electrical engineering at the University of Pennsylvania and graduated from Jefferson Medical College before completing his medicine and cardiology training at Mount Sinai Hospital in New York City. Prior to starting the Prevention and Treatment Clinic at North Shore, he was on the full-time faculty of Columbia University's medical school in New York.

Over the last year, Dr. Bernstein has presented research at the annual meetings of the American Heart Association, the American College of Cardiology and the Heart Failure Society of America and at programs sponsored by hospitals such as Johns Hopkins, the Winters Center for Heart Failure Research at the Texas Heart Institute and Albany Medical College. He has lectured at the European Heart House, the InterAmerican College of Cardiology, the Canadian Cardiovascular Society, the International Society for Heart Research and the German Society for Prevention and Rehabilitation of Cardiovascular Disease.

He participated in the creation of treatment guidelines for Action-HF and the Heart Failure Society of America for the treatment of heart failure. Dr. Bernstein is currently a member of the Clinical Cardiology Council of the American Heart Association, the Heart Failure Society of America and is a Fellow of the American College of Cardiology.

Much of his research focuses on patients with heart failure, an advanced form of heart disease. He also has helped run international trials of heart attack treatments. His current research focuses on the treatment of fatigue in people with heart disease.